Best CARE Best FUTURE

A Guide for
HEALTHCARE LEADERS

||||||||||||||||||||||||||||||||||||||||||||||||||||

David M. Lawrence, MD

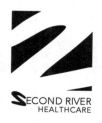

SECOND RIVER
HEALTHCARE

BEST CARE
BEST FUTURE
A Guide for Healthcare Leaders

Second River Healthcare
A Healthcare Leadership Publishing Company
26 Shawnee Way, Suite C
Bozeman, MT 59715

Phone (406) 586-8775
FAX (406) 586-5672

Copyright © 2014 David M. Lawrence, MD
Editor: Tiffany L. Young
Cover Design: Lan Weisberger – Design Solutions
Typesetting/Composition: Neuhaus/Tyrrell Graphic Design
Editing Style: The Chicago Manual of Style – Sixteenth Edition

Lawrence, David M.
Best Care, Best Future: A Guide for Healthcare Leaders / David M. Lawrence, MD
ISBN-13: 978-1-936406-20-3 (hardcover)
ISBN-13: 978-1-936406-21-0 (softcover)
ISBN-13: 978-1-936406-22-7 (e-Book)

1. Healthcare Leadership   2. Innovative Healthcare   3. Patient-Centered Care

Library of Congress Control Number: 2013951951

First Printing   February 2014

Innovative Health Speakers, a speaker's bureau and division of Second River Healthcare provides a wide range of authors and nationally recognized experts for speaking events. To find out more, go to www.InnovativeHealthcareSpeakers.com or call (406) 586-8775.

Second River Healthcare books are available at special quantity discounts. Please call for information: (406) 586-8775 or order from either website:
www.SecondRiverHealthcare.com | **www.BestCareBestFuture.com**

"He saw his job as managing the disruptive process of devising and implementing a new system. [...] He needed to provide hope without raising expectations that were unrealistic [...][And] he needed to allow a measure of stability in employment and daily life even as the system underwent fundamental changes."

Ezra F. Vogel
Deng Xiaoping and the Transformation of China

TABLE *of* CONTENTS

Praise for:

BEST CARE, BEST FUTURE:
A Guide for Healthcare Leaders

This is a well-written, easy-to-read book by a "Hall-of-Fame" healthcare leader. But it is much more than that. It is full of ideas and insights that are worthy of study and reflection. The author describes what an action leader does and then self-critically observes those actions in order to learn and change himself and his organization. Everyone in health and medical care should read and study this book. Leaders in all walks of life will find that the leadership ideas apply to them.

Paul O'Neill
Seventy-Second Secretary of the US Treasury

David Lawrence provides a must read for today's healthcare leaders intent on ensuring their organizations endure and thrive in a rapidly changing environment. He draws upon decades of personal experience and astute observation to create a guide to navigating large scale change in an industry that has historically been change averse and now must change at warp speed.

Gary S. Kaplan, MD
Chairman and CEO
Virginia Mason Health System
Seattle, Washington

BEST CARE, BEST FUTURE is truly a must read for all healthcare executives. David Lawrence has put together what will become the playbook for individuals tasked with leading and transforming our healthcare system. In a very practical approach replete with great examples from Kaiser as well as other health systems, this book will certainly become the go to book for those of us trying to help right America's healthcare system.

David Feinberg, MD, MBA
CEO, UCLA Hospital System
Associate Vice Chancellor
UCLA Health
Los Angeles, California

From start to finish, Dave Lawrence's book is compelling and instructive. Dave is a renowned leader and his stories, vision, and practical strategies provide insight for today's healthcare leaders preparing their organization for success in the future. The book should be required reading for all leaders.

Maulik S. Joshi, DrPH
President, Health Research & Educational Trust
Senior Vice President of Research
American Hospital Association
Chicago, Illinois

Dr. David Lawrence's new work is a candid, clear, and compelling handbook for leading change. Lawrence takes us inside the mind of great leaders and provides us with morally based, practical wisdom that is grounded in deep and raw experience. Lawrence delivers actionable advice for navigating in uncertain times. Don't be fearful of the future. Learn from the best.

Ian Morrison, PhD
Healthcare Author, Consultant, and Futurist
Menlo Park, California

A seasoned captain of healthcare transformation, David Lawrence provides a credible guide to navigate the permanent white water of today's healthcare environment. With a heading set to continuous improvement, *BEST CARE, BEST FUTURE* maps out the roles of leadership, partnerships, and systems that ensure a safe arrival for the best care possible to all the patients we serve.

James A. Diegel, FACHE
President and CEO
St. Charles Health System
Bend, Oregon

As the latest version of the healthcare reform unfolds, serious concerns about the rapidly rising cost, as well as uncertainty about quality, safety, and value signal that change is inevitable this time. There are few historical precedents for the kind of disruptive change that will be required to right our healthcare delivery system. However, in *BEST CARE, BEST FUTURE*, David Lawrence, informed by his depth of experience and refined notions of leadership, offers a frank and discerning "guide" for healthcare leaders embracing change. Offering uncommon clarity, Dr. Lawrence lays out a formula for the kind of healthcare leadership necessary to transform our healthcare delivery system—founded on ethical values and not about authority or title, but about influencing outcomes and inspiring others.

Michael L. Steinberg, MD
Chair of the Clinical Chairs
UCLA Health
Los Angeles, California

In *BEST CARE, BEST FUTURE*, David Lawrence has created the most direct and powerful account yet of the challenges of leadership in transforming healthcare. Drawing on a decade at the helm of the largest private nonprofit health system in the United States, Kaiser Permanente, he uses front-line accounts of difficult decisions, mistakes, and hard-fought wisdom—always tempered with humor and generosity—to argue the case for leadership that puts patients at the core of every decision.

Molly Joel Coye, MD, MPH
Chief Innovation Officer
UCLA Health
Los Angeles, California

A wonderful read—wise, human, and honest. David's leadership stories and defined building blocks are a Master's guide for improving care delivery.

Diane Cecchettini, RN
President & CEO
MultiCare Health System
Tacoma, Washington

BEST CARE, BEST FUTURE gives us something few other books do; theory in the hands of a master practitioner. Drawing from the literatures on leadership and healthcare, and his own extensive experience, David Lawrence provides counsel to healthcare leaders, both new and seasoned. With advice that is both specific and detailed, he gives a frank description of the challenges healthcare leaders face—personal and practical—and how to deal with them. In an era when calls for leadership in healthcare are both commonplace and vague, Lawrence's clear description of the job of leadership, and his guidance to how to do it well, is a breath of fresh air.

Richard Bohmer
Former Professor of Management Practice
Harvard Business School
Boston, Massachusetts

International Visiting Fellow
The King's Fund
London, United Kingdom

This is a very thoughtful book. It beautifully uses anecdotes and personal experience to get across the concept of leadership. Most importantly, Dave Lawrence lived it before writing it. He shows leadership is earned, one mistake at a time.

The most useful chapter is on leading what some would say are the unleadables—the physicians. But, as Lawrence makes admirably clear, that just isn't so. That chapter is one of the best, all illuminated by stories with relevant messages and a strong moral core.

John Horty
Chair, Estes Park Institute
Managing Partner, Horty Springer & Mattern

Changing the way care is organized and delivered is the central challenge facing the US healthcare system today. We desperately need leaders who recognize this and have the courage to take the controversial steps necessary to change course. That is why Dr. David Lawrence's book *BEST CARE, BEST FUTURE: A Guide for Healthcare Leaders* is so timely. I recommend it to anyone who believes in better health, better care, and lower cost.

John A. Kitzhaber, MD
Governor
State of Oregon

Transforming delivery of medical care is to the twenty-first century what sanitation was during the Industrial Revolution—the greatest health challenge of its time. This book provides a hands-on guide for leaders who aim to drive their organization toward a vision of delivering what David Lawrence calls "the best care possible" every day, day after day. It is an honest and wise reflection of a great leader who understands the challenges he describes because he lived them—been there and done that—before creating organized systems of healthcare delivery was recognized as a moral and competitive imperative. Among the core messages he imparts is to maintain the centrality of patient experience in order to motivate change. Reading this book feels like having your own professional coach and mentor near at hand. Leaders of healthcare organizations should read it, keep it on their bookshelves, and refer to it often.

Sara Jean Singer, MBA, PhD
Associate Professor of Health Care
Management and Policy
Harvard School of Public Health

Department of Medicine, Harvard Medical School

Mongan Institute for Health Policy
Massachusetts General Hospital
Boston, Massachusetts

Dr. Lawrence's lessons from his tenure at Kaiser are refreshingly candid and insightful. Everyone who aspires to be a twenty-first century healthcare leader should take heed to his guidance: partner with your patients to design care, cultivate self-awareness, and avoid the "shiny objects" that distract you from your primary responsibilities; and surround yourself with the best team possible to achieve your goals, regardless of whose interests may be jeopardized. The leaders we need will find or discover the best-known care possible for their patients, and acknowledge that when they fail to lead their organizations toward this goal, they are responsible for the harm that is inflicted as a result. Every practice leader at Massachusetts General Hospital will receive a copy as soon as this is published!

Susan Edgman-Levitan, PA
Executive Director
John D. Stoeckle Center for Primary Care Innovation,
Massachusetts General Hospital
Director, Massachusetts General Hospital
Primary Care Leadership Academy
Boston, Massachusetts

FOREWORD
by Richard J. Umbdenstock

Calls for visionary leadership in healthcare are in no short supply these days. Consumers, payers and purchasers, policy makers and providers themselves, share the urgent need to change the course of our healthcare system in pursuit of long-term sustainability. What is in short supply, however, is agreement on what that system vision should be, the ability to communicate the vision clearly, and the understanding of what it will take for the leader of a healthcare enterprise to guide the organization toward its vision while remaining viable along the way.

As I returned to the AHA in 2007 as its president, I attended a retreat where a colleague offered an important element of that vision from the delivery side of the equation. He said, "We must build a system where the expertise of the physician is reserved for the point of clinical ambiguity." What a simple, if not eloquent, observation. I've carried it with me through the ensuing debates over things like payment formulas, scope of clinical practice, continuity of care, and team-based care. For me, that observation has been a gift.

The observation came from David Lawrence. David is not only an experienced clinician and integrated care executive, he is someone with a gift for clarity of both vision and word. And this "guide," as he humbly calls it, is his most comprehensive gift to our field.

As we charge into a future that we already know will be more integrated organizationally, more at-risk financially, and more accountable publicly for results, we very much need the experience and distillation that David provides. The value in having David's lifetime of experience lies not just in knowing more about the organizational characteristics of Kaiser Permanente, with its integrated clinical and financial functions, it lies in hearing what it took inside the organization to build a functional learning system that has the financial and performance risks to strive each day to unlock the next best answers of effectiveness, efficiency, teamwork, and service.

In this piece, David offers many more elements of a coherent vision on, for example, continuity of care ("A successful system connects illness care and daily life through clearly marked bridges that help patients move back and forth depending on needs and medical conditions.") and equity of care ("If you've ever been sick in a country whose language and culture is not yours, you know how difficult it can be to get the care and the comfort you need.") Moreover, there's advice on the principles and practicalities of effective leadership of others and of one's self, of organizational structures, and management techniques. And there's the added benefit of observations from his pursuit of learning in corporate boardrooms and executive suites inside and outside of healthcare that few in our field have had the chance to experience.

But maybe the greatest contribution of all lies in part three, where David explores seven basic systems that constitute a "robust operating system [...] systems [that] create the context, the soul, the meaning for what the organization provides, and how it operates." Few authors in my experience, whether consultants or practitioners, have been able to pull these elements together in as coherent and helpful a manner.

Books need a target audience; those that have something for everyone often spread their focus and dilute their impact. In this case, practicing healthcare leaders will all find parts of this guide helpful, but it will be helpful in different ways to different leaders depending on where they are on the organizational and personal journey. For existing CEOs, the discussion of starting out new in a leadership role may seem too late to be helpful—maybe—but not if one admits that the transformation called for means they must become the new CEO of an entirely new organization. For others, there may be no more important chapter than the one on exiting and transitioning as a leader who ensures a level of continuity, and opportunity, that is so important in the cycle of on-going organizational evolution and re-creation. For particular audiences—boards, medical staffs, other members of the leadership teams come to mind—there may be some sections that are more helpful than others as these groups seek greater insight into specific aspects of the complex world of healthcare leadership. And for sure, this entire piece will become an invaluable text for those early careerists who want and need a well-constructed and comprehensive reference piece to use as a touchstone for career design and development as an organizational leader.

Healthcare has been blessed by many talented and dedicated leaders, and it has been my privilege to have known and learned from so many. Each has been a gift in some unique way—whether it was their particular strength in facilitating consensus in a room full of highly opinionated individuals, in envisioning a new and better system of care to deliver higher and ever improving quality for the sake of our patients, or in motivating needed behavior changes through changes to the payment systems. I wish each of them could have written down their lifetime of experiences and perspectives as a contribution to those who will build on their success. In this case, I am extremely grateful that David Lawrence has done just that. No one has seen more of the future than David through his pioneering work in integrated and accountable care. And no one could have put it all together in a more eloquent and humble fashion.

Richard J. Umbdenstock

President and CEO of the American Hospital Association

FOREWORD
by Donald M. Berwick, MD, MPP

The Knife Edge trail is a famous approach to the summit of Mt. Katahdin in Maine, and a dangerous one. Over a mile long, it narrows to less than three feet wide for hundreds of yards, with drop-offs of several thousand feet on each side. Only serious hikers need apply.

The Knife Edge came to mind when I first read David Lawrence's book. A leader, like David, in a time of big change walks a perilous, narrow path. He may see further than many others—that, in fact, is part of his job—and so must point out hazards and unpleasant facts of life that many do not yet see (and frankly, do not want to see). And yet, he knows that engaging those threats successfully is possible only with the full-hearted investment of talent and energy from those led; they cannot be forced or required to do that, only their authentic choices matter. No leader in a complex, human endeavor can succeed *through* the people (let alone *despite* them), but only *with* the people.

It is a narrow trail between the despair, fear, and anger of people receiving unwelcome news and the power of people fully able to resist and paralyze action. That's the problem: "Deliver the tough facts, and nonetheless win their hearts and minds."

David Lawrence assumed leadership of Kaiser Permanente at a time of big change. KP is without a doubt one of the great American institutions of the twentieth century. At its founding, it represented a breakthrough in design and conception about the relationships among people who receive healthcare, people who give healthcare, and the financing and management functions that make their interactions possible. It became the wellspring for the modern movement toward integrated care. My decades of work in the field of healthcare improvement have included a continual search for innovations and successes that could be studied and spread. It has seemed to me that, no matter what problem we were addressing—asthma care, obstetrical management, waiting times, heart failure management, prevention, end-of-life care, patient education, and on and on—with stunning regularity we could find somewhere within KP one of the best models in the nation, if not the world. To call KP successful is a vast understatement.

And yet, like every other healthcare organization in America, KP found itself in rough waters as the twentieth century began to close, and faced a challenge of identity and strategy if it were to become fit for the twenty-first century. Those were the challenges that David Lawrence took on as the new leader. And so, he found himself on the Knife Edge. How could he tell his colleagues in one of most successful organizations in the history of modern healthcare that the old way could not be the new one, and yet retain and build upon the pride and joy in work that, alone, could carry KP into its own future? It wasn't easy.

This book tells that story. With his immense intellect and perceptiveness, David redacts his own story into specific and memorable lessons, captured here in lists and models of principles, practices, and checklists for leaders. These will be invaluable guides for those who, like David, must help organizations navigate change. Keep your notebook by your side as you make your way through the book; you will want to remember these teachings.

But these pragmatic lessons, useful though they are, are not for me the most memorable part of this master's lesson. Instead, what I find most remarkable of all is David's own confession of his vulnerability and personal transformation as he tried hard to understand how to tell the unwelcome truth and yet win the will of his colleagues, freely given.

His account of this change comes early in the book, and he introduces it with these words:

> "Feedback was consistent from my senior team, outside
> observers, people throughout the organization, and my
> coaches: I had locked myself in a bubble as the voices
> around me grew louder, more unpleasant, critical, and
> sometimes personally insulting. I was less and less will-
> ing to listen to people who disagreed with me, and often
> rejected ideas at odds with my own."

Thus did David's most important leadership journey really start. And thus did David encounter afresh the third of the leader's great tasks. The first task is to see and tell the truth, unwelcome though it may be. The second task is to realize and submit to the fact that only the freely given will and energy of the workforce can produce success; that there is no real power worth a damn beyond that. The third task is to know oneself. And the third is the hardest.

Generations—maybe millennia—have built the myth of the leader who knows, without doubting self, the problems and the solutions. And leader after leader, I think, has suffered from hiding the painful secret of not knowing and yet claiming to know. My great friend and mentor, Paul Batalden, once drew me a diagram of the pathway of organizational transformation and put at the top—Box #1—the words, "leaders' curiosity."

To lead well, one must be willing to become vulnerable, uncertain, and curious. In this book, David Lawrence tells of such a personal transition directly and courageously. It is a lesson to be learned that underlies all of the valuable lists and diagrams he also generously offers.

Learn this from David: never, ever try the Knife Edge alone. To cross it safely, you will need the humility to go with others, to tell them you are afraid, and now and again to reach out your hand to another to steady your step. It is in your willingness to accept your own vulnerability and to ask for and embrace help that you will find your true leader within, as David Lawrence did.

Donald M. Berwick, MD, MPP

Former President and CEO
Institute for Healthcare Improvement

Former Administrator
The Centers for Medicare & Medicaid Services (CMS)

ACKNOWLEDGMENTS

This book owes its life to many, though I am responsible for its content.

Michael Steinberg: for introducing Jerry Pogue and me

Jerry Pogue: for guiding this book from start to finish

Tiffany Young and the team at Second River Healthcare: for untiring support and excellent editing

Don Berwick, Maureen Bisognano, Molly Coye, Jim Diegel, Gary Kaplan, Ian Morrison, Rich Umbdenstock, and Paul O'Neill: for friendship, support, and ideas; and for pointing me to leaders who are making a difference today in healthcare delivery

Richard Bohmer, Molly Coye, Jim Diegel, Maulik Joshi, Al Jubitz, Jeff Parker, and Sara Singer: for reading early drafts, and providing helpful insights and invaluable critiques

Diane Cecchettini, David Feinberg, Loo Choon Yong, and Eugene Washington: for giving me a front row seat as you wrestle with the challenges of delivering healthcare in the twenty-first century

The many healthcare leaders in the US and elsewhere: for giving generously of your time, and for patiently explaining how you strive to deliver the best possible care every day, day after day

My friends and colleagues at Kaiser Permanente: for your friendship, support, and devotion to giving our patients and members the best care possible

Robert J. Mignone, MD, my brother: for giving each patient your best for nearly fifty years, and for never ceasing to improve what you already do so well

SPL: for your love, strength, and example

Our children and grandchildren: this book is dedicated to you. In some small way I hope it can help you receive the best possible care each time you need it.

PREFACE

In 1957 I shipped out on the SS Columbia Trader, a Liberty ship that carried surplus grain from Portland, Oregon to Pusan, Korea. When we neared the coast of Japan, we slowed, then drifted, engines idling. A typhoon lay ahead, so the captain ordered us to store equipment, lock down hatches, tighten lines, and secure the doors and portholes in the main cabin to prepare the ship. Hours later we moved through the Tsugaru Strait between the islands of Hokkaido and Honshu into the Sea of Japan. All the next day we hugged the coastline of Honshu heading south along the edge of the storm. Still the seas were heavy. The ship shuddered as we plunged into the huge waves that broke over the bow and swept past the steering cabin high above the main deck. By early evening the storm veered away from us, the sea calmed, and we made our way safely to the small seaport city of Moji, Japan, to refuel before going on to Pusan.

We were fortunate. Later that fall a different crew returning to Korea on the same ship ran into a huge storm off the Aleutian Islands. The captain chose to ride it out, but the ship was too slow and heavily loaded, unable to adjust easily, its steel fatigued from countless trips back and forth across the Pacific. After hours battling heavy seas, a large crack opened across its body. The US Coast Guard responded to the distress call in time, and towed the ship to a nearby harbor for emergency repairs. Once these were completed, the ship limped back down the coast of North America, up the Columbia River into the Willamette River to dry dock in Portland.

We face major storms in healthcare. How long they will last is anyone's guess. Should we become an Accountable Care Organization? Should we buy physician practices? Build a primary care network? Join others in a larger network? What will the new state insurance exchanges in the Affordable Care Act mean for us? How can we reduce our costs to keep our margins acceptable in a world of shrinking reimbursements? Can we hire and retain qualified nurses? How do we compete against independent ambulatory treatment centers established by community physicians? Should we accept bundled payments and other at-risk payments, or remain in the fee-for-service business as long as we can? How can we avoid re-hospitalization penalties and take advantage of the other pay-for-performance opportunities? How do we reduce our costs without destroying our balance sheets and compromising our quality? Can we really achieve the Triple Aim (Bisognano and Kenney, *Pursuing the Triple Aim*)? The questions never stop. Unknowns multiply. The water seems to get rougher, the waves higher. More storms lie ahead as far as we can see. What can we do to survive? What is our safest course? How do we prepare our organizations to navigate safely through what we face now and what lies ahead?

This book is intended to help you answer these questions. What can you do to improve your chances of survival? And how can you change your organization to get there? It is written for leaders of healthcare delivery organizations, but the recommendations are relevant to anyone in a leadership position regardless of your role or the size of your organization. The recommendations apply equally to leaders in the US and those in other parts of the world because care delivery and medical practice vary little from country to country, and the storms are similar wherever we look.

My experiences, good and bad, both inside and outside healthcare, inform what you will read, and insights from many colleagues have further shaped my perspectives. At the outset be assured that I do not ask that you become Kaiser Permanente, or any specific organization for that matter. Far from it. Your answers will grow from your needs and realities. As the tennis star Arthur Ashe once said, "Start where you are. Use what you have. Do the best you can." (Forrest Calico, with Joyce Sweeney Martin. *Out of the Blue*, 2012)

Every leader of a healthcare delivery organization has three responsibilities. First is to ensure that each patient, each consumer of the services, and each community served receives the best care possible: the safest, most effective, timely, responsive, efficient and equitable care we know how to provide today. It is the care that improves the quality of life of the patient, lowers the costs of care and improves the health of the communities we serve. The leader is held accountable to this standard in law and regulation, and makes this promise to those who depend on the organization for their care. It is a legal and moral obligation, our bedrock commitment as leaders.

The second responsibility is to build an organization that competes effectively. This means generating the strongest margins possible to invest in growth and provide the tools for twenty-first century medical care, while delivering superior care and services that meet the needs of the populations you choose to serve. If you happen to be a for-profit delivery enterprise, it also means producing economic benefit for your shareholders. A leader's third responsibility is to prepare the organization for the future, to ensure that the people, the values and mission, the systems, the culture, and the financial resources are sufficiently strong and coherent for the organization to navigate through whatever storms lie ahead.

As we consider how to respond to these obligations, we face a serious dilemma. To meet our responsibilities by continuing our current course is the comfortable alternative, what we know, familiar territory. We are blessed with well-trained professionals and, compared to the rest of the world, unequaled technologies and infrastructure. Yet the weaknesses in today's models make this a dangerous choice. We tolerate large variations in clinical care from physician to physician, and from episode to episode of care. Physician autonomy inhibits care coordination and performance measurement, and adds waste to our care processes. After more than a decade of work, preventable medical errors still cause unnecessary suffering, even death. Our services are often organized for the convenience of the providers instead of the patients and healthcare consumers. Escalating costs collide with shrinking reimbursement levels to narrow operating margins. Although we know these things, our models are difficult to change, slow to adjust, ponderous like the Columbia Trader, fatigued from fighting the day-to-day battles of care delivery.

Anyone who has tried to change a care delivery system knows the risks, has experienced firsthand the furious resistance and how slowly the direction shifts. Our traditions and cultures are powerful, reinforced by decades spent navigating through blizzards of traditions, unwritten rules and explicit requirements, as well as ethical and moral constraints, social expectations, community demands, laws and regulations, and always changing technologies. We are reluctant to abandon the security and safety of what we know, and worry that the new will drive out what is right about what we do now. Most of us would prefer a slow, cautious path if we agree to change at all. And all of us wonder how we will fit in and what will sustain us after we change. Those who think they will lose fight harder *against* the changes than those who might gain fight *for* them.

Yet we face demands and unknowns that force us to look for another course. Plunging ahead with an organization and culture ill-suited for the storms we now face is the riskiest choice we have. We must look for an alternative. No course is easy or risk-free. There is no silver bullet. And our challenge goes far beyond simply choosing a different route. We have to change our direction without capsizing our organizations, and we need to build new capabilities to undertake the journey. This guide is intended to show you what that course is and how to navigate such a change successfully. But let me warn you. This is a long journey. It will take years. You cannot turn a key or wave a wand to make it happen. You cannot buy a solution off the shelf. It is hard and arduous work for you and those you lead. It takes unwavering will and courage.

We must start with a clear view of our destination. In my mind, it is simple: *superior quality, the best care possible.* Our goal must be to eliminate every preventable error that can cause harm or death; provide only care that is effective, that matters to the patient, when the patient needs it; and provide all care without waste or prejudice. We seek to help every patient get better (or as "well" as our science permits) consistent with his or her values and wishes, reduce costs to the lowest possible level, and help our communities be as healthy as possible.

Care is everything that happens to a patient from the moment she expresses a concern until she receives the best possible response and experiences the best possible outcome. It is much more than an exchange between one provider and one patient. Care includes all the interactions between physician and patient, as well as all interactions with other clinicians and support staff. It involves the transfers, the information, the studies, the images, the flow from one step to the next. To reach our destination we must learn to fit these pieces together, integrate every element for each patient and for all patients into a larger, well designed, coherent process, in other words, a system. It also involves what happens before an individual seeks care from the formal medical care system: what community she lives in, how she cares for herself and her family, and what kind of environment surrounds her.

And we can never reach our goal. Ever. Our understanding of the science of medicine is always changing, the tools and technologies available to us continue to improve, our insights into the needs of our patients, consumers, and communities shift, our understanding of what works and what doesn't continues to evolve, and our competitors never stand still. The conditions we work in constantly shift too, the politics, the demands of payers and consumers, the demographics of our nation, the availability of trained healthcare workers and physicians. We are in the middle of many storms and will continue to be for as long as we can imagine. Superior quality always changes, the bar always rises. Like the Fountain of Youth, our destination is a dream, a mirage. We are always becoming.

If we never get there, why do it? Simply stated, the journey itself is the important thing, our unending search for better answers, our obsession to deliver superior care for every patient every time, our unceasing hunt to discover the best "what" and "how" of care delivery. These are the capabilities we must build. Yet we are not used to always becoming in healthcare. We prefer to settle on what we consider the best solution now and stick with it until forced to change. Routines help us avoid mistakes and remember critical steps, after all. We might claim to be data-driven learners and scientists, but in truth we are creatures of habit. Our challenge as leaders is to create and sustain a kind of institutional schizophrenia: on the one hand ensuring the stability we need to deliver superior care each day, while at the same time living in a state of perpetual discovery and change to find what is best for our patients and communities.

Why is superior quality the preferred destination and the search for it your safest course? Most importantly it's the right thing to do. It is hard to argue that we can do anything less. Beyond the moral imperative, there is an equally powerful business case for undertaking the quality journey, especially in healthcare. Care quality determines in large measure whether or not patients and communities place their trust in you and, as a result, choose you and your physicians when they have another alternative. It determines whether or not you can hire and retain the best physicians and nurses, the best clinicians, a dedicated support staff, and principled, high integrity senior leaders. It determines how expensive your care is to deliver, because almost without exception, better care lowers your operating costs. As a result, it is an important hedge against eroding reimbursement rates, and helps protect your balance sheet and long-term financial strength as well. Finally, to deliver ever-better quality, your organization must learn to adjust, change, and drive forward in the face of resistance. This capacity is your compass and gyroscope, it both guides and balances you as you seek the safest passage through the unknowns that lie further ahead. In a word, this course offers the greatest likelihood that you can meet your responsibilities as a leader.

Like the preparations a crew does to protect a ship and its cargo before heading into a storm, making sure that the quality of care you provide today is as good as possible is the first step in your journey. But to do this again and again, to constantly learn and change and improve, to innovate and invent, you have to do much more than a one-time fix. You start by being honest with yourself about what is important to you, what you stand for, believe in, what you are capable of in terms of leadership, and what capabilities you need around you. Leading a change in course like this demands more of you than you have ever given before. You need a solid foundation, your own deep moral core, to lead this way. Only then can you build strong, resilient partnerships with key constituents inside and outside your organization, including with those you serve. Finally, you must establish the systems that help you steer the organization on the course you and your partners have selected: the system of language that shapes and molds the conversations, the mission, the values, the purposes, the tactics, the successes and failures as you move forward; the systems of learning and transparency that reinforce the importance of experimentation, challenging, and a "no secrets" culture that can use data and information effectively to make course corrections; the information systems that provide the data you need to track your course and plot your future route, as well as link together caregivers and patients and the organization itself; the innovation system that helps you discover and extend discoveries into the daily work of providing and supporting care; the system of prods to help you keep your organization on course; and the system of accountability and compensation that reinforces what is important and rewards the successes. To shape these partnerships and systems into an engine that is powerful enough to drive your organization through the storms toward its ultimate destination requires a unifying operating discipline that is up to the challenge—robust, reproducible, analytic, detailed, and, above all, proven.

The book is organized to reflect these requirements. In the introduction, I describe some of the changes we made at Kaiser Permanente between 1991 and 2002, and the challenges we faced in doing so. My intent is to show you that you really can do what this book recommends.[1] For the reader interested in an in-depth exploration of that period or of KP

[1] The reader interested in an in-depth exploration of that period or of Kaiser Permanente (KP) itself may wish to review the Kaiser Permanente Oral History Project at the Bancroft Library at University of California-Berkeley.

itself, I refer you to the Kaiser Permanente Oral History Project at the Bancroft Library at University of California-Berkeley. In part one of this guide you will find several chapters designed to help you lead. In the first three I explore basic questions: *"Why is a change of course necessary?"*, *"What does the new organization look like?"*, and *"What kind of leader do you have to be?"* The section concludes with chapters about how to start your tenure as a leader, the obstacles and traps you can expect to encounter, and how to protect your personal health as you take on a challenge like this. In part two we examine the partnerships you need to take your organization in its new direction. These start with the most important of all, your "partnership" with the patients and the communities you serve. Then we shift to the board of directors, your senior leadership team and change leadership team, the physicians, and the workforce. I conclude with an exploration of compacts, a vehicle for formalizing and focusing these relationships, and for assuring that they endure through the inevitable ups and downs that will occur. In part three, we examine the systems you will need: language, learning, transparency, innovation, and information; the prods; and the accountabilities and compensation program you put in place to reinforce the changes. In the final chapter, I discuss how to integrate these capabilities with a robust operating system to drive your organization on its new course.

This is a guide not a memoir. Of course I draw upon my experiences—successful and unsuccessful, inside Kaiser Permanente and out—to highlight many of the recommendations. After the introduction, you will find only short anecdotes, usually at the start of the chapters or sections, and italicized so you can skip over them if you prefer. Occasionally I cite a journal study or a specific quote in the text. In the bibliography are references that have informed my thinking for the book and influenced my own leadership journey. In appendix A is a summary of the recommendations you will find throughout this guide. In appendix B are the names of the individuals who generously shared their perspectives with me in preparation for the book.

You will encounter the term "patient" again and again. I use it to include the patient who seeks care, the consumer who wants services unrelated to a specific illness, and the families who support both. A separate consideration is the term "community," a placeholder for any community your organization serves. I have used the feminine pronoun "she" throughout the book because it is simpler than saying "she or he" each time, and reflects the majority of the healthcare workforce, including younger generation physicians, in the twenty-first century.

You will also note that this book concentrates on how to change healthcare delivery organizations. Largely unexplored is how these organizations fit into the larger mosaic that influences and shapes the health of individuals, communities, and even nations. This is intentional. How to improve the health of our populations, how to change the many institutions that influence our health, how to shape and inform the individual behaviors that contribute to overall health...these are pressing questions that lie beyond the scope of this guide. Instead I have focused on the question of how to deliver medical care more effectively, and how to change the institutions, the systems, and the organizations that provide medical care.

Importantly, you are not alone in your search for the best route through the storms, and you can join with others to learn what may work. You may be part of a larger system that can make the identification and sharing of the best care solutions part of its work (see, for example, the Care Management Institute at Kaiser Permanente described in chapter eighteen, or consider the role of NICE with the National Health Service in the UK). You can join innovation networks to identify care enhancements more quickly. The Institute for Healthcare Improvement has provided extraordinary guidance and support for more than twenty-five years. National organizations like the Health Research & Educational Trust (HRET) share care delivery insights, as does its parent, the American Hospital Association (AHA). A host of other national organizations support hospital executives and medical leaders as well. You do not have to be a lone ranger.

It takes courage and skill and unrelenting will to undertake the journey described in this book. Before we explore how you can meet the challenge, let me assure you that I am not asking you to do the impossible.

INTRODUCTION

"...our life is not our life, merely the story we have

told about our life.

Told to others, but—mainly—to ourselves."

– **Julian Barnes**, *The Sense of an Ending*

IT CAN BE DONE

Kaiser Permanente doesn't change easily. It wasn't designed to. Care is delivered by physicians who belong to their own "Permanente" medical group. They elect their medical director who serves at their pleasure, as do the chiefs of departments, and the clinical directors of each clinic and hospital. At one time there were twelve such medical groups within Kaiser Permanente, each with its own medical director, board of directors chosen from the partner physicians, legal charter, and contract with the local Kaiser Foundation Health Plan and Hospitals organization. "Kaiser Permanente" is a partnership of these Permanente Medical

Groups (PMGs) with a single, national entity called Kaiser Foundation Health Plan and Kaiser Foundation Hospitals (KFHP/H). Much of the power, many of the decisions, and all of the clinical care are in local hands.

The governance of Kaiser and its physician partners makes change even more difficult. Paired with the leadership team of each medical group are executives of the Kaiser Foundation Health Plan and Hospitals (KFHP/ H) organization. These KFHP/H executive teams report through the national CEO of KFHP/H to the independent board of directors of the KFHP/H Corporation. To comply with laws in a few states, several regional KFHP/H organizations have been organized as subsidiaries of the parent entity with their own local board of directors in addition to the parent board. All KFHP/H corporations are not-for-profit, 501(c)(3) community benefit entities with specific responsibilities, limits, and benefits spelled out in both state and federal law.

Leading each region is a senior executive (regional manager) and the local medical director. As noted, these partners make most decisions for their region, independently or together, depending on the issue. In the past, regional managers, medical directors and a handful of national officers, including a representative for the PMGs, established Program policies and national strategic direction through the so-called "Kaiser Permanente Committee," a group of more than thirty members that met three times each year. Between meetings, national decisions were brokered among key players, typically the leaders of the two large California regions, the national officers, and any other regions that had a stake in the issue. When they did occur, organization-wide agreements were crafted in a time-consuming, consensus-building process that moved back and forth between the regions and the national organization until an acceptable solution was found.

For more than forty years this structure worked well. By 1991, a total of 8,674 full-time physicians were employed by the twelve PMGs to care for 6.5 million members in sixteen states plus Washington, DC. In addition to these physicians, Kaiser Permanente employed seventy-five thousand people, of whom 75 percent were members of one of thirty-six unions operating under more than fifty separate labor contracts. The Program owned and operated twenty-six hospitals and over two hundred ambulatory centers. Annual revenues that year were $9.831 billion. The two California Regions accounted for two of every three members, physicians, and employees in the Program. Kaiser Permanente had become the largest private healthcare system in the world. It has been described as a super-tanker, but this understates its massive scale and labyrinthine complexities.

When the board of directors of Kaiser Foundation Health Plan and Hospitals appointed me as CEO in 1991, they challenged me "...to prepare the organization for the twenty-first century." Between 1991 and 2002, we successfully changed our course. We weathered difficult controversies as we tried and failed, started again, learned, adapted, and slowly built important new capabilities over those eleven years. People joined at all levels to shape the solutions that have become part of today's woodwork. It was hard work and it took time, and through it all, we remained true to the traditions and core values that had already brought us so far.

In the first few years our focus was to improve performance in each region. After extensive debate in the Kaiser Permanente Committee, we agreed that substantial changes were required. We adopted a "Quality Agenda" designed to achieve cost-savings, competitive advantage, and long-term strength through care quality improvement. The Kaiser Permanente Committee delegated authority for leading this work to a small leadership group that included, among others, the executives of the two California regions and medical groups. And, for perhaps the first time in Program history, we engaged outside experts to help us.

Five years later we had little to show for our investment. Regional teams conducted extensive studies to understand their competitive challenges and opportunities for improved performance. But the local leaders balked once they saw how extensive the changes would have to be. It would take years to persuade the physicians and other clinicians and support staff that these changes were in their best interests and those of their patients. We had started at the wrong place.

Although the studies had little impact on regional performance, they profoundly affected the board of directors of KFHP/H. As we monitored the results and responses, a clearer understanding of important weaknesses in our decentralized model emerged. We noted the wide variations in quality and operational practices from region to region. Good ideas rarely traveled from one region to the next because of the strong "not invented here" culture. Every region designed and built its own hospitals and ambulatory facilities. Each region had its own IT solution, with a unique platform, vendor relationships, staffing, management, and oversight arrangements. Most had initiated their own electronic medical record solutions. We could not leverage our massive scale to purchase goods and services at favorable prices. Finally, the laborious consensus-building decision process among our many constituencies made it difficult to respond to the growing number of opportunities and threats we encountered.

Complaints from our national customers reinforced these concerns. They demanded greater consistency among the regions, and warned us that our competitors were better able to meet their needs than we were. To make matters worse, malpractice litigators had begun to exploit differences in care from one region to the next to bolster their arguments.

By midway through the decade, the senior team of KFHP/H and the board reached an important decision. To provide the best care possible to our members, our patients, and our customers, we had to become a more cohesive national program. We needed a different balance between the physician and KFHP/H organizations, as well as regions and the national program. But this new capability, we knew, had to rest on the bedrock principles and long history that had contributed so much to the success of the organization.

Late in 1995, we took the first step. We placed virtually all information technology-related funds in the Program into a single national budget managed by a newly recruited national chief information officer (CIO) in KFHP/H. A steering committee was created to represent the KFHP/H regional leadership, the PMGs, and the national offices, chaired by a senior physician executive from the Southern California Permanente Medical Group. The CIO, together with this committee, was given responsibility for developing the IT strategy for the Program and regions, proposing budgets for the approval of senior management and the board of KFHP/H, and overseeing the implementation in collaboration with regional IT leaders. Within a few months, the CIO and steering committee, working with regional representatives from the medical groups and the KFHP/H organization, conducted an extensive review of the existing electronic medical record initiatives, chose the best among them, and provided a detailed budget and plan for extending that solution to the entire Program. When the board approved the recommendations, the decade and a half-long effort to connect the entire organization with a single EMR solution began. (See chapter seventeen.)

Later that year, we took several more actions. PMG leaders must always weigh the interests of their own medical group against those of the Program as a whole. Most concessions to the collective interests reduce their degrees of freedom to lead their own individual group. Not surprisingly, we could make little headway when we discussed matters of national concern with their national representatives, and our group meetings with the medical directors on these subjects were time consuming and largely unproductive. So we stopped meeting this way and sought the views of the individual medical directors directly in one-on-one discussions. We also made several organizational changes and replaced two respected senior KFHP/H regional managers. As difficult as these decisions were to make, they were even harder for the organization to accept. Criticisms of my leadership grew. Morale plummeted. One medical group, I was told, actively explored whether or not to secede from KP and establish an independent health insurance plan to compete with us.

Even so, the Program's instinct for self-preservation kicked in. PMG and KFHP/H leaders formed a small group to redefine the relationships between the two sides of the organization, and after several months, produced a new compact that detailed the commitments of each to the other. A key provision included a streamlined national leadership group with representatives from the medical groups and KFHP/H that would provide strategic guidance and clarify common purpose for the organization. The agreement codified the respective decision "rights" of the PMGs and KFHP/H, and reaffirmed that partnership-based cooperation remained a bedrock principle.

During that same period, the PMGs created the Permanente Federation to provide a coordinated voice for themselves. They chose a trusted medical executive, J. Francis "Jay" Crosson, MD, as the first president and delegated important responsibilities to him and his team. Less than a year later the Federation chartered the Care Management Institute (CMI), responsible for developing and implementing national clinical standards across all the medical groups. While the Federation represented a major shift in thinking for the PMG leaders, the decision to build the Care Management Institute meant that, for the first time, the individual medical groups ceded responsibility to a national body (which they "owned") to create the standards and tools to practice more effectively and efficiently, and help them realize their goal of delivering superior care throughout all their medical groups. (For more detail about the CMI, see chapter eighteen.)

As we closed out the year in 1996, we had started to build important new capabilities. We still had a long road ahead, of course, but it looked like we were on our way. Then the bottom fell out.

In the first five quarters of 1997 and 1998 the Program lost more than $500 million; the first losses in our history. Our credit ratings fell, and we faced a serious liquidity crisis. A concerted effort on the part of some leaders to return to the old ways of doing things threatened to undermine the changes we had been able to make. Compounding the disarray, the CFO of KFHP/H resigned for personal reasons. And the medical directors asked the board of directors of KFHP/H to fire me.

They argued that I had created turmoil in the organization by challenging our traditional culture and values. Moreover, in 1997 I had supported a zero premium increase for the third straight year. They were right on all counts. The organization was destabilized. We had challenged ourselves. And I did believe that we had learned to control our costs well enough to justify another zero rate increase. I was wrong. Our membership growth overwhelmed our hospitals and emergency rooms, and forced us to contract for care outside KP at exorbitant prices. This, together with an unexpected (and unprecedented) rise in hospital utilization rates across the US, created the perfect storm that nearly capsized us.

The board, though, was committed to our course and rejected the request to replace me. But they made it clear that they expected me to right the ship financially and address the morale problems as quickly as possible. They wanted results.

We were able to stop the bleeding after five quarters. Dale Crandall, an outstanding financial leader from outside healthcare, joined us as CFO and reestablished our lines of credit, patiently explained our financial situation inside the organization and out, and put us on solid financial footing once again.

In the midst of that financial crisis, we concluded a two year negotiation with twenty-five of our twenty-six AFL-CIO union affiliates to create a national labor management partnership that enabled us to work more collaboratively in teams across the entire organization. It remains the largest such partnership in any industry in the US (see chapter eleven).

We seemed to be back on track, but to realize the full benefits of the changes we had made, I needed a better way to lead. Many people, especially in the medical groups, struggled with the changes. My decision on rates had precipitated our financial losses. Physician leaders had demanded my resignation. Some experiments, like combining the KFHP/H regions in Northern and Southern California, worked poorly. We were only just emerging from years of labor turmoil. I knew I couldn't be successful if I continued as before.

Feedback was consistent from my senior team, outside observers, people throughout the organization, and my coaches: I had locked myself in a bubble as the voices around me grew louder, more unpleasant, critical, and sometimes personally insulting. I was less and less willing to listen to people who disagreed with me, and often rejected ideas at odds with my own.

Despite the controversies inside the organization, I was in the spotlight outside of it; I was sought out for my opinions and often asked to speak to leaders in other organizations. But as those outside demands grew and the unrest inside the organization escalated, the information sources so crucial to understanding the issues and getting feedback dried up. My lines of communication into the organization were more limited, the reach of my contacts shorter, and the information increasingly filtered through the small cadre of people around me. Instead of direct, regular, and informal conversations, I heard mostly what my leadership team thought was important. I had started to believe my press instead of facing my strengths and weaknesses head-on.

I also knew that I had to broaden my approach to decision making. In the early years, I had used the traditional channels and relied on our time-honored consensus approach to change our course. It hadn't worked. To make the important changes we needed, I'd made unilateral decisions instead. Now I had to find a path that lay somewhere between these extremes in order to develop better solutions for the issues we faced going forward, and build greater support for the changes we had to make.

Gradually, with good coaching, I improved. It wasn't easy, but I began to seek dissenting views again. I listened with greater patience and less defensiveness, and tried to incorporate the rhythms and needs of the organization, the outside pressures, and the important responsibilities that KFHP/H had to those we represented into my decision making. Jay Crosson, a steady, thoughtful influence throughout the time we worked together, was an invaluable partner.

Successes started to come more frequently. We completed the closure of four regions that had lost money for at least a decade. This difficult process required trust and collaboration among the leaders of the individual PMGs, the Permanente Federation, and the KFHP/H.[2] Our important Community Benefit Program was retooled as well. Although legally the responsibility of KFHP/H, that effort had been a long-standing source of pride across the entire organization. We had always included a wide range of local and national efforts under its umbrella, but we faced growing challenges from state and national legislators who

---

[2] In 2013, the Program leaders announced the sale of the Cleveland Region reducing the number of regions to seven.

sought to redefine our community benefit obligations more narrowly than we thought appropriate. In 2000 Jay Crosson and I established a joint KFHP/H and PMG work group to formalize a more coordinated national community benefit effort and to create an explicit annual Program funding target. Once the proposal was approved by the KFHP/H board of directors, that same group wrote the job description for a new senior vice president to lead the implementation, then recruited, interviewed, and recommended three candidates for Jay, the medical directors, and the senior team of KFHP/H to consider. Raymond J. Baxter, PhD, accepted our offer and immediately set about transforming our community benefit program. Today the organization invests approximately $2 billion per year in community benefit efforts, the most notable of which are directed to improving the health of underserved communities throughout the states served by the Program.

Occasionally, I still acted unilaterally—in patient safety, for example. From 1998 to 2000 I participated in the Executive Session on Medical Error and Patient Safety at the Harvard Kennedy School. Leaders from healthcare, government, and the media met several times a year to review the growing literature on patient safety, discuss ways to address the problems from a policy perspective, and share the experiences of our organizations. Five of us, all CEOs of large healthcare organizations, held monthly phone meetings to discuss our progress and commiserate about the obstacles we encountered. All were actively pursuing a patient-safety agenda in their systems, convincing me to do more in ours. It was slow going. KP leaders were worried about greater public scrutiny and potential legal exposure, and the physician leaders were concerned that a focus on medical errors implied that they and their colleagues were doing something wrong. Some questioned whether or not we had a patient safety problem in the first place.

As the speaker at the National Press Club luncheon in July 1999, I chose to focus on patient safety. Several participants from the Executive Session helped me prepare. The press reaction was positive. Inside the KP Program the response was less enthusiastic, but within a short time the medical directors and Dr. Crosson created the National Patient Safety Committee chaired by Michael Leonard, MD, an anesthesiologist from the Colorado PMG (whose courageous story about his own medical error appeared in *The New York Times* later in 1999). KFHP/H representatives were included in the committee, and, as a result of their work, patient safety innovations began to move across the Program, medical errors were reported more regularly, practices from other systems were introduced into KP, and our safety leaders became active in national patient safety efforts outside the Program. Today KP is one of the leaders in the nation's patient safety movement.

During the period between 1991 and 2002, we added important new capabilities to the Program. The Care Management Institute and the Labor Management Partnership allowed us to leverage the wisdom of physicians and employees across the Program for the benefit of all our patients and members. The Permanente Federation and the national leadership group balanced the historic strength of the regions and provided new vehicles for reaching alignment on key strategic matters throughout the Program. Innovations moved more easily from region to region as traditional boundaries gave way to greater cooperation. Decisions were made more rapidly. Systems were established to take advantage of our scale as a purchaser and supplier. We began the long road to connect clinicians and members with a comprehensive electronic medical record and communications system, and in the process, lay the foundation for a remarkable database to support future studies of care quality. Considerable influence still remained with the regions, and the Permanente Medical Groups were legally and functionally independent as before. But our traditional building blocks were balanced by new Program-wide capabilities that could help us take advantage of our unique scale and experience, bring greater cohesion to the organization as a whole, and provide better care to our members, our patients, and our customers.

Our performance reflected our growing capabilities. Revenues in 2002 were $23 billion, up from nearly $10 billion eleven years earlier. Our net income approached $1 billion. Though we had reduced the number of states we served from sixteen to nine (plus the District of Columbia) when we closed the non-performing regions, our membership reached 8.5 million, and the Permanente Medical Groups employed twelve thousand full-time physicians to care for them. Our regions received high ratings from the National Committee for Quality Assurance (NCQA) and other national bodies. With a strong credit rating and balance sheet, and a growing reputation for quality and patient safety, we were well positioned for the future.

The changes were not easy, and it would take several more years and new leadership to stabilize the organization. But we were now ready for the new century. We had successfully changed our course. As the guide that follows shows, so can you.

PART ONE

PREPARING TO LEAD

In 1913-1914 former President Theodore Roosevelt and the Brazilian adventurer, Col. Candido Rondon, explored the Rio da Duvida, River of Doubt, in the Amazon basin of Brazil. The river was uncharted. It ran hundreds of miles through deep jungle against the Eastern slopes of the Andes where few outsiders had ventured before. The two men, Roosevelt's son, and their crew navigated the length of the river, but suffered deaths, major illnesses, injuries, and near starvation in the process. Of the nineteen men in the original party, sixteen survived. The leaders had anticipated a different experience. Dugout canoes designed for the calm waters of the lower Amazon broke apart in waterfalls and rapids. Most of the men, Roosevelt and his son included, contracted malaria. Natives were dangerously hostile. Roosevelt never recovered and died five years later.

We have much more to go on in healthcare than Roosevelt and Rondon did on their adventure. We are not talking about unexplored territory. Others have changed the course of their organizations. A rich literature exists about change and leadership. We know how and where to find the best care possible. We don't face a River of Doubt. The stakes are high, but we are unlikely to suffer injury or death as a result. We know what to expect and can prepare for what lies ahead.

And preparation is crucial. You may have moved into your leadership role from managing an operational or functional area. Perhaps you shifted from a leadership role in a smaller organization. No matter what you have done before, leading an organization through a major change is different. You need new skills, new approaches, a deepened sense of what you believe in, and what is important to you. You don't want to waste valuable time getting up to speed, and you want to avoid mistakes if you can. People in an organization watch their leader carefully, especially so when you are starting out. Their first impressions, and the stories they create about them, are hard to change. You want to be more right than wrong from the beginning because as a leader you don't get many "do-overs."

Your preparation begins with a reflection on what you do in healthcare, why you do it, and what you believe and feel most deeply about as a leader. You also want to examine what you have learned and what you believe about leading others. You need to review your successes and your failures, and the strengths and weaknesses of leaders you've known and of the organizations you have visited. Read and visit all you can. Develop your own clear-eyed assessment of your capabilities and those of your organization: strengths and weaknesses, and the changes needed to thrive in the future. Together these insights form your internal compass that guides you as you lead others through the changes ahead, your "true north," that provides focus and fuels your passion. You will return here again and again to regain perspective and quiet distracting voices, to find the will and courage to persevere.

Your private stories help you make sense of why you need to change the organization, what you need to change it to, and how you intend to get there. The stories you share with others create the common ground, the glue, for collective purpose and direction, and passion. Whether private or public, they must be palpable, real, and living; they have to ring true. You find them in the voices of the people you serve and those who take care of them. You find them, too, in your own experiences. They broaden your lens, sharpen your focus, and deepen your perspective. You have *to watch out for tools and words that separate you from these voices, which make people smaller and distant—like looking through the wrong end of a telescope. Be careful of statistics and what Don Berwick, the founder of the Institute for Healthcare Improvement, has called "distance-words": disease burden, prevalence, incidence, patient satisfaction, worker engagement, and even quality, safety, efficiency, or discharge and compliance. You must not insulate yourself or your organization from what real people go through to get care, the confusion they feel when care doesn't work for them, their fear when ill or injured, and their uncertainties when different physicians tell them different things. You must not hide from what professionals and support staff go through to do their work, their doubt and shame when things go wrong. You must not hide from yourself either. Used without thought, statistics and distance-words obscure the essence of what you must understand and feel to make sense of what you hope to do and why.*

As important as stories are, your preparation requires much more. You have to plan for the issues that affect your ability to lead. How will you engage the organization as you begin? How will you prepare the soil for your eventual departure so the changes continue after you leave? What obstacles are you likely to encounter and how will you deal with them? What traps await you as a leader and how will you avoid them? And finally, how will you protect yourself—your personal health and your energy—throughout this long change process?

CHAPTER ONE

WHY CHANGE?

My mother died at age ninety in her own bed. She was free of pain and fear and fully conscious until hours before her last breath. The day before she died, the head of housekeeping and the hairdresser at the retirement home stopped by to share the latest gossip. Earlier in the week she read stories to her great-grandchildren gathered on her bed. In those last weeks, my brother, sister, and I reminisced with her about our life together. We cooked her favorite meals. A nurse's aide helped her with her personal needs. We held her as she died. As these things go, it was a good death.

Getting there was a different story.[3] Like many her age, she had several chronic conditions. Until four years before her death, though, she was active and in reasonable health. Then she fell leaving an evening meeting, broke her leg, and damaged her shoulder. Her downward spiral accelerated after that, and the dangerous flaws in her medical care became obvious.

She was taken by ambulance to an excellent community hospital that was part of an "integrated delivery system." The following morning

---

[3] This experience is described in more detail in a "narrative matters" article for *Health Affairs* published in 2003. "My Mother and the Medical Care Ad-Hoc-Racy." *Health Affairs*, March 2003, 22:238-242

her leg was surgically repaired by a well-regarded orthopedic surgeon, and after three days, she was transferred to a good rehabilitation facility nearby. There she spent more than three weeks mostly waiting: for her medical records to arrive from the hospital; for her dermatologist to return from vacation and make his treatment plans for her skin cancers available to her other physicians and the rehab facility nurses; for the rehabilitation physician and the operating orthopedist to coordinate her physical therapy; for the home care service to get back to the rehab center to agree on follow-up therapy; for her oncologist to write treatment orders for her slow-growing lung cancer; for the nurse's aides to figure out how she might exercise when she couldn't use crutches with her damaged shoulder; for the chief nurse and the night nurse's aide to agree on whether or not she should get up to toilet or use the bedpan at night. In the four weeks from her fall until her release from the rehab facility, she was cared for by ten physicians, at least fifty nurses, ten physical and occupational therapists, and a host of nurse's aides. Her stay at the rehab facility was more than twice as long as anticipated. By the time she returned to the step-down unit at her retirement home, she was angry and frustrated as a result of the mixed signals, poor communication, and conflicting information about her future.

She never fully recovered. She made several trips to the emergency room after that, most of which resulted in another hospital admission, further work-ups, more tests, different treatments, and a never-ending parade of new physicians, nurses, and therapists, each with her own approach. Finally she had had enough. She was tired and ready to die.

Unfortunately, her primary care physician thought she was depressed and refused to authorize hospice care for her. When we were finally able to reach Mom's oncologist, he signed the orders. The first session between Mom and the hospice nurse lasted more than an hour as they talked about her care and her wishes. Care unfolded like this from then on. Mother was the center of attention. She took part in almost every discussion and decision as long as she was able. In the hours and days she had left, her caregivers made sure she was able to sleep when she wanted to, free from pain, and without shortness of breath. She was *mentally alert, and as warm and funny and loving as always until she lapsed into a coma hours before her death.*

Mom was part of a good delivery system with a good reputation. Its physicians were some of the best in the city. Its hospitals were well regarded. The rehabilitation program was top-notch. The management was motivated and ethical. All the pieces were in place: a network of hospitals and nursing homes, relationships with community-based physicians, even an electronic medical record system in their hospitals. They presented a common "brand" to the community. They arranged contracts with several insurance plans. They purchased many goods and services for their hospitals through a central purchasing office. A single board of directors oversaw the system and hired and evaluated the CEO. They published data about their care that showed reasonable performance on common quality and safety statistical indicators. But the care they provided was fragmented and confusing. The system leaders had neglected their most important responsibility: to put the pieces together and organize the care itself.

Each physician did her best. So did each nurse and health worker. The hospital and rehabilitation facility were modern and pleasant. The technologies were up to date. But hand-offs were fumbled, important information was lost or unavailable, and treatment plans were poorly coordinated. There were delays and conflicting diagnoses and treatments. Decisions were made without Mom. She didn't know why her care failed to make her better, she worried that it was unsafe, and she was angry that it reduced the time she could spend with her family and friends.

This is not an unusual story; Mom's care is similar to what many people receive, especially those with complex or chronic conditions. The individual professionals and support staff are usually good; the resources are usually acceptable. But the care is not integrated or coherent. There is no specific path for the patient to move from start to finish through the system to get what she needs, no plan that makes sense of the recommendations of each individual clinician, little collaboration among clinicians, and no overarching purpose or shared values to create an integrated whole.

We need competent, well-trained, and ethical physicians, nurses, and other health workers. Our buildings must be well designed and safe, the technologies we use effective and safe too. But this is where care systems often stop. They assemble the pieces and hope for the best. To provide the best care possible consistently, these elements must be integrated into a coherent care process that works for the patient.

Had Mom been cared for this way, she would have joined her physicians and other clinicians to design her personal care plan. The home care, physical therapy, pain management and wound care specialists would have participated too, offering their experience and expertise, and their insights from conversations with Mom. Together this team would have decided how to match the best available practices with Mom's wishes. They would have shared information electronically throughout the process regardless of who provided the care, where it was delivered, or when it happened. No matter where she went, everyone would know her, and her clinical information and important personal information would move with her. She would know how things worked too: how to get her questions answered, where to go to resolve a confusing conversation, and how to be sure her medicines and her care were safe. She'd know these things because the clinicians and the support staff would give her the information, and because the system itself would provide IT and phone portals where she could get answers to her questions and find the clinical information she wished to have. She would have been involved every step of the way because she and her family would have the information needed to help her make decisions consistent with her needs and values. She would not have wasted time getting her care either; unnecessary steps in the process would have been eliminated, her progress through the system orderly, and simple. Throughout both the acute phase of her accident and the ongoing care she received in those last four years, the physicians and nurses and others would have reviewed her status regularly in order to change the plan as needed, identify where improvement could occur, and determine how they were doing compared to the expectations they had established ahead of time. They would have checked up on her at home between regular visits and before she needed to go to the emergency room. The management of the system and the board of directors would have reviewed the same data, not to interfere with the clinical discussions between the clinicians and Mom, but to ensure that everyone, including themselves, met the quality standards they all had agreed to. If Mom's care had been designed this way, the outcome may not have changed very much, but the care would have been far better for her and far less expensive for those who paid for it.

CHAPTER TWO

WHAT DOES THE NEW ORGANIZATION LOOK LIKE?

It looks familiar. Physicians and nurses, other clinicians, support staff in and out of exam rooms or hospital rooms. Patients surrounded by their families. The smells and sounds. Monitors blinking and beeping. Modern technologies. In the hospital or the ambulatory care center, the clinic or the physician's office, you feel right at home. Look more closely, though. Talk with patients and physicians and the people. This is a different organization than you are used to. It isn't perfect. There are always ways to get better. Everyone seeks to improve by finding ways to work more effectively and efficiently. They don't give up. They never stop. What makes them this way? How did they get this way?

To provide the best care possible requires an ecosystem that supports constant change and unending improvement. In the chapters that follow, we explore what that ecosystem looks like and how to build it. But first let's consider its major features. First, it has bridges that help patients move between their medical care and their broader lives. It recognizes that the best care occurs when the best of medicine joins with the best social support systems. Next, it recognizes that the quality of its care depends on both care process and care content. Its people focus on how to improve the way patients move through the entire care process, as well as the specific care they receive at each step. Third, it is relentlessly collaborative. Teams and groups care for the patients and work together to understand and improve the care they provide. Fourth, it improves and innovates at a faster pace than most care systems can. Finally, it is coherent. Its people know what they want to be, how to get there, and are unyielding in their drive to get there.

Bridges

When you are a patient, your care begins with a concern, an accident, or a question, and continues until either the best possible solution is found, your life returns to as close to normal as possible, or you reach the end of your life after everything you want done has been tried. During this process, the patient usually interacts with the formal "illness care" system and the physicians or nurses, pharmacists, and clinicians who work in it. Sometimes that involves a relatively straightforward episode of care—a knee replacement, for example. Sometimes, as in a chronic illness, it can occur again and again. The patient moves back and forth between her daily life and the system and clinicians who provide her medical care. No system can provide everything the patient needs to have the best outcome. The patient relies on her family and friends, sometimes on people who have experienced the same problem or have the same question, and sometimes on resources from the community. Neither the care system, the patient, her family, nor the community around her can do it alone. They have to work together, and this requires bridges.

A patient with stable, insulin-dependent diabetes, for example, may make six physician visits in an average year. While there, she may have blood work done, or an imaging study or two. She may go to the pharmacy to fill a prescription. Each "episode" might involve as much as an hour of interactions with health professionals. That's six hours of formal care a year. Even if these interactions take two hours each time, the patient will spend only half a day a year in the formal care system. You get the idea. The other 364 ½ days a year, she's on her own. She has to figure out how to conduct her life, take her medications, manage her diet, control her weight, carry out her work, maintain her social life and her family, and keep her condition in check. Her success depends in part on getting the right combination of insulin. But she's in charge. She monitors her illness to decide how to modify her daily insulin based on what is going on in her life that day, and to be sure no complications have arisen that require attention.

Providers may say, "We've done our part, now you are responsible. Come back and see us if you need more care from us." When we think this way, we can convince ourselves that the patient is "non-compliant" if she gets sick again or develops complications. We may shrug these complications off as "inevitable" with an illness like this. We provide the medications and the education, after all; the patient is responsible for what she does with it. If we do what we're supposed to do and the patient does what we advise her to do, everything would be great. But we know this is not the best care because it disconnects the clinicians and care system from the lives of their patients, from what the patient must manage to achieve the highest possible quality of life.

A successful system connects illness care and daily life through clearly marked, easy-to-use bridges that help patients move back and forth depending on needs and medical conditions. A common approach is to simplify access to the clinicians: easy appointment making, including online services through system-sponsored portals, simplified telephone appointment making, large blocks of unscheduled physician and clinician appointment time for walk-in and same-day appointments, call-lines staffed by nurses and sometimes even by physicians. Navigation support programs help patients get to the right clinicians or follow-up appointments. Before patients leave the system, they are connected to community resources where they can find emotional support, answers to their questions about how to manage their daily lives, where to find goods and services they require, transportation to help them get from one place to another, home-maker services, or meals-on-wheels if they are disabled or elderly. If patients live in rural areas where access to specialty care is difficult, or if they have difficulty with personal mobility, electronic and video consultations connect the patient with her primary care clinician or other treating specialists. A growing number of patients use in-home monitors to collect and send clinical information to their caregivers and their clinicians about their status. Often this helps the patient remain at home or at work, make necessary treatment and lifestyle adjustments, and avoid a trip to the hospital or clinic.

Bridges like these join the care a patient receives from the illness care system to personal and community sources. They are integrated to produce the outcomes the patient seeks instead of forcing the patient and family to figure it out on their own in the never-never land between the recommendations of the formal care system and the world they live in.

Solid bridges require sound footings. In healthcare this means a clear understanding about what you contribute to the patient's health and well-being and what the patient's life and circumstances contribute. The greater your understanding of the resources in the community, the tools and support systems available, the needs and challenges a patient faces in living her life away from your formal illness system, the more robust your care will be. Instead of a moat that separates your care system from the lives of your patients, you want bridges that are open all the time and have few obstacles to their use.

When it comes to bridges, a particularly difficult design challenge is the construction of primary care services, where your formal illness care system most often connects to the broader lives of your patients and communities. You may believe you need relationships with primary care providers to support your specialty care services. Or you may provide comprehensive medical services through networks, contracts, or even ownership of primary care providers. Whatever your rationale, the traditional delivery model is physician-based, even the emerging "medical home" models. Here's the rub. There are not enough primary care physicians in the pipeline to meet the projected demands of our growing, aging, and increasingly diverse population, and the deficits are projected to increase over the coming two decades at least. The gap won't be filled with nurse practitioners, physician's assistants, or foreign medical graduates either. You are not likely to be able to find enough physicians or physician-substitutes to provide primary care the way we have in the past. Even new physician-based delivery models may not be able to meet the demands. The numbers don't add up. You are probably going to need different solutions.

But what an opportunity this presents! Access barriers (lack of insurance and limited physician availability) and crowded emergency rooms are forcing people to find other ways to obtain the primary care solutions. Services once provided by the physician, nurse practitioner, and physician's assistant are now available on a mobile phone or over the Internet. Advances in molecular science (genomics and proteomics especially) enable more precise diagnosis of diseases before they become symptomatic, and understanding of risks that can be moderated through changes in lifestyle. Distance diagnosis and treatment, even remote robotic surgery, enable patients to bypass local provider systems. New competitors have emerged to provide some elements of traditional primary care: screening, triage, treatment of simple acute illnesses, management of medications and complications that are medication related, and navigation support. Some are based in retail spaces.

Because primary care is in a state of flux, patients have access to a growing array of choices and are likely to have many more in the coming years. While this is a significant opportunity for those who can take advantage of it, the solutions are not self-evident. You would be wise to experiment with different primary care models and with different linkages into the communities you serve. You might establish a formal innovation program directed to this goal, funded and managed as part of your ongoing efforts to serve your patients and maintain your position in your markets. (See chapter sixteen). You may encourage more spontaneous innovation in new forms of primary care delivery with recognition programs, early-stage support, and the like for both individuals and teams within your system. At a minimum, you need an intelligence-gathering group that is charged with keeping track of developments in primary care that could have value for, or pose threats to, your current organization.

Process

A system that provides the best care possible has an obsessive focus on how patients can move efficiently and safely through their care process. Every step is designed to support what occurred before and what comes next, and fits into the overall puzzle. Every step is considered in relation to all others in the process. There is a smooth, transparent flow from the moment a patient enters the system to the moment her dependence on the system ceases. Different conditions require different processes, so within any care system many solutions will run in parallel to accommodate the variety of patients you serve.

The steps are linked in different ways. The most obvious is information that travels with the patient so everyone involved knows what happens all along the stream. But connectivity is only the start. The people involved—the physicians, nurses, other clinicians, and support staff—determine ahead of time how their patients will move from step to step, and decide what must occur at each step. They review the evidence to decide what the condition requires and they agree in advance how they will make their decisions. They design the entire process to be as efficient and effective as possible, both for the patient and themselves. They combine a comprehensive view of the entire process with the detailed design of each step required to move from start to finish through that process.

They also anticipate how to care for the patient who doesn't fit the mold, when something additional is required or something unplanned occurs. For any given condition, the design may include several branches, an "if-then" approach to accommodate these situations. But what of the uncommon? Here, too, contingency plans are required. They define how to recognize when the common approaches don't apply, and what to do instead. They determine in advance who needs to be involved in such situations and how. Care is designed, planned in advance, and takes into account the fact that patients don't always fit perfectly into the expected mold. Options and contingencies are built-in. You start by designing for the patients whose care is relatively predictable. Then you plan for the known variations that occur in a smaller number of patients. Finally you design for how you will deal with the exceptions where the solutions must be tailored to a unique and unusual situation.

Understanding and designing the patient's flow through the system, then, is a central focus. Without this, it is impossible to stabilize, let alone measure and improve what occurs. This attention to the process and content of the entire experience recognizes that care is a product of myriad interactions and actions that must be integrated to produce the best outcome. The best care is delivered through a carefully constructed process, not a series of independent interactions.

To stabilize flow and the decisions that get made throughout that process requires the clinicians and support staff to replace their traditional idiosyncratic approaches with standardized solutions wherever possible, and with defensible variation where the science and experience do not support a single approach. Theirs must be an unrelenting quest to reduce variability throughout the care process and in the content of care. The limits to variation reduction are determined by the science and collective wisdom of your clinical colleagues. And there must always be a fail-safe when a patient requires care that lies outside these limits. Physicians and other clinicians must be able to pull the cord for the exception. They must be able to make the difficult clinical judgments for that subset of patients who require them.

Picking one way to do things is often controversial. Physicians resist "cookbook" medicine even as each uses her own to manage her patients; exceptions can be found for most rules. It helps to distinguish between defensible variation in a clinician's approach to diagnosis and treatment, (where the science and collective experience does not support a single solution for all situations), and the selection of standard procedures for the multitude of steps in care that do not affect clinical decision-making but are part of the process of getting care. Most steps in a care process can be standardized, both in their sequence and in what occurs at each step. We see this in everything from the way a patient is admitted to a hospital, to the way information is collected and initial studies are performed in an ER, to the way a patient moves through a physician's office for a routine visit. We see it in the imaging suite, where technicians follow standard procedures for most of the studies they carry out. And we see it in the way instruments are sterilized and packed for use in the OR suites. The list is endless.

You want to standardize as much of the patient experience as possible, and as much of the support required for that process as you possibly can. The closer to standardized your care processes and content are, the easier it is to design the flow from step to step, measure whether or not the care is delivered as intended, and adjust the expectations in light of new information. It is also easier to train everyone as to what is expected: it doesn't take as long, is less expensive, much safer, and more reliable.

Diagnostic and therapeutic decisions lend themselves to standardization, but only up to a point. Whenever physicians and other clinicians can agree on what information they need for every patient in order to establish the diagnosis and initiate the treatment, this reduces the likelihood that critical steps will be skipped, duplicate studies will be done, or critical communications between the staff and the patient will fall through the cracks. It is even better if the clinicians can agree on the criteria for how to integrate historical, physical, laboratory, and imaging studies to make a particular diagnosis or initiate therapy. However far the evidence can take you, the goal is to agree ahead of time how care will be provided. You want to exhaust all possibilities for standardization and variation limits, consistent with safe and effective care, before you default to the exception, rather than assume every patient requires a customized solution. They don't, and they suffer needlessly when a system functions this way. Variation should widen as the clinical problem becomes more obscure or complex. It needs to because this is where the evidence is weakest and the problem-solving ability of the physician, especially the specialist and sub-specialist, comes into play. What is going on and what to do about it may be a dilemma, or it may require a series of special tests to figure out. The evidence doesn't support tight limits in variation, and certainly not a standardized solution. But the steps a patient goes through to get to this point, the process required to obtain the necessary information and tests, may be the same as every other patient with that general kind of problem (cardiovascular, neurological, etc.). The only way to know is for those involved to review the evidence and their collective experience to see how far they can go in standardizing or agreeing to boundaries before they default to the customized solution the patient requires. The framework Christensen, Grossman, and Hwang provide in *The Innovator's Prescription* (2008) is useful. The authors differentiate the routine clinical problems from the most difficult and ambiguous ones that require unique solutions. In these situations, they argue, the best care occurs when specialists join the patient and family to determine the appropriate solution and build the appropriate plan. They call these "solution shops," and argue that complex clinical problems require shared problem solving—a combination of minds and experience—rather than the serial referral from one specialist to the next as in the past.

You also want to standardize across conditions and situations wherever you can. You can simplify administrative processes and information gathering and processing, for example. Utilities within the system—the IT system, the laboratory, and the imaging service—can have standardized processes for accessing, registering, recording, and reporting that cover most patients. The process is exactly the same as within a given condition or general problem area: array them side by side to see where they are the same or similar, modify them as far as you can to achieve a standard approach across them, and continue this until you exhaust all possibilities and further standardization is not possible.

Collaboration

A hallmark of high performance is collaboration. Clinicians must work together, with support staff, and with patients and their families to determine what is best for any given patient. Physicians can no longer act autonomously and provide high-quality, twenty-first century medicine; they have to work together to find the answers they seek. This means a change in the traditional hierarchical relationships among the healthcare professionals. Instead of the physician always assuming control, care decisions are shared among the physicians and other clinicians, and sometimes the support staff, working collaboratively with the patient and family. Team-based care, either face-to-face or virtual, requires flexible leadership and greater collegiality than you might be used to. Better solutions emerge when clinicians share their insights with one another and when a group of clinicians, support people, the patient, and family work to find the best answers.

This is a far cry from the "cowboy" that Atul Gawande describes in his provocative *New Yorker* essay "Cowboys and Pit Crews." To be a high-performing system means you confront that tradition of autonomy and control head-on. Collaboration is essential. Medical science and medical technologies far exceed the ability of any one physician or clinician to manage alone. The more complex the patient, the more crucial it is for different clinicians with different areas of expertise to share in the care. Referring the patient is not sharing, however. These patients require discussion, exploration, and weighing of choices. They need the insights of all the clinicians to get the best care. The recommendations must be synthesized into a coherent plan of care that fits their values and their situation. People need to talk together to do this; it can't happen one referral at a time.

This is what you want to create. You want groups of clinicians talking with patients and their families about what is going on and what to do. You want clinicians to gather around the patient's bed to make sure everyone is on the same page each day. You want physicians and nurses and other clinicians to talk to each other by phone, iPad, or video conference when they cannot meet face-to-face. You want to see time in the daily schedules for these gatherings to occur. And you want everyone involved to review the work to make sure yesterday's decisions still apply today given the information at hand. You want to see collaboration.

The absence of shared information and discussions like these, the persistence of silos in which each physician does her best based on what she knows without the insights of the other physicians and clinicians involved, means more errors and harm because the decisions don't fit together. They are not integrated. When the patient and the family have to figure it out alone, it is a recipe for trouble. Collaboration is a central tenet in twenty-first century medical care. Medicine is too complex and too dangerous to practice any other way. The ethical commitments that physicians and other clinicians agree to when they enter their professions require it, while at the same time, they retain responsibility for maintaining their individual competence as professionals.

Speed

Speed is not something often associated with healthcare organizations. We are conservative and careful; change occurs slowly, even reluctantly. We demand data and more data. Internal politics must be carefully navigated. But successful systems have learned to speed up this process. By outside standards they would hardly be considered "speedy," but in the context of healthcare they certainly are. They attack the issue head-on, recognizing that they must keep improving, keep innovating to stay current if they are to provide the best care possible to those they serve. They have learned to make incremental changes again and again, analyzing each change carefully, then making adjustments, then analyzing, and adjusting, in that ongoing cycle of continuous learning and improvement. They understand that no change is permanent; all changes are temporary; learning is constant, as is improvement. The changes in these more advanced systems come faster and more readily than in others precisely because they have created an ecosystem to support these faster learning and innovation cycles.

Coherence and Constancy

The final characteristic you need is a shared sense of purpose and direction throughout your organization. People have to know what they intend to create to deliver the best care possible, why, and how they will do it. This coherence is more than a shared view of the future. It also includes the values that guide the organization, how you treat one another and especially patients, and the ethical framework for your work. This is rarely perfect. Not everyone understands; people don't always use the same language. But it is what you strive for. You want everyone to be able to describe how they contribute to the purposes of the organization, and cite examples of behaviors that reinforce those values and purpose. The other piece of this puzzle is the determination, the drive throughout the organization to get it "right." It is an obsession. Your people need to search for the best solution they can find now, then relentlessly make it better and better. That journey defines the organization—its purpose and its work.

Does all this matter? Will an ecosystem with these characteristics change your performance? There is no overarching measure to distinguish the best from the rest, no side-by-side study that compares performance across systems. But there are compelling indications that a system with these characteristics delivers better care.

The strongest case is that a handful of healthcare systems and a wide range of companies in other industries have built ecosystems like this, and driven their quality to the highest levels observed in their industries. Companies as different as Intel, Agilent, McKesson, Singapore Airlines, and Toyota, for example, are well known for operational excellence and their obsession with reliability and safety. They continuously make improvements to increase the performance of their goods or services, and to drive out waste; they innovate through their efforts and the companies they purchase to expand their capabilities. They produce best-in-class results, including financial strength, and have done so for many years.

Impressive results have been reported by the highest performing care delivery systems in the US and elsewhere as well.

In the February 2013 issue of *Health Affairs*, CEOs of several leading health systems described how they have reduced costs by raising quality. This article is an outgrowth of work these individuals carried out under the aegis of the Institute of Medicine to create a CEO Checklist for High-Value Health Care as the report is called (Institute of Medicine, 2012).

Denver Health has had the lowest reported observed versus expected mortality ratio among the nation's academic medical centers for the past five years running. They also have the lowest severity adjusted maternal mortality rates in their labor and delivery service in the state of Colorado, a position they have held for the past five years as well.

The UCLA health system moved from the thirtieth percentile to the top ranked academic medical center in the nation in overall patient satisfaction in less than five years.

ThedaCare reports that their average "door-to-balloon" time for treatment of myocardial infarction has dropped from around seventy minutes with wide variation to thirty-seven minutes with narrow variation in three years as a result of continuous improvement in their intake and screening processes in the ER.

Working together, representatives of Intel, physician leaders in Washington County, Oregon, and the back specialists at Virginia Mason Medical Center reduced the cycle time for patients with back injury from fifty-two to twenty-one days. Ninety-six percent of patients received evidence-based diagnosis and treatment; patient satisfaction reached 98 percent, as did same day access for care. One hundred percent of patients returned to work. And there was an estimated 10 to 30 percent savings in time for patients who participated in the redesigned value stream compared to those who did not. (Bisognano and Kenney. *Pursuing the Triple Aim*, 2012)

The Urban Health Institute at Mt. Sinai Hospital and Health System in Chicago worked with community leaders and families to reduce the frequency of childhood asthma in several target communities by improving the ability of families to care for their children. In a two year period, hospital utilization declined 81 percent, hospital days 69 percent, emergency room visits 64 percent, and urgent care department visits 58 percent. (Whitman, et al, *Urban Health*, p. 260)

At Intermountain Healthcare, quality leaders summarize their work over two decades in the *Health Affairs* article "How Intermountain Trimmed Health Care Costs Through Robust Quality Improvement Efforts." For example, leaders there report a reduction from 28 percent to less than 2 of clinical inductions for labor that failed to meet strong indications for clinically appropriate inductions. Similarly, the caesarian section rate at Intermountain is reported at 21 percent versus the national average approaching 34 percent.

At Long Island Jewish Health System, the search for the best care possible begins and ends with patient involvement. Patients and their stories are throughout their hospitals. The culture of patient centeredness permeates the organization, and is a core building block for the new medical school that the system has created.

The Norton Health System in Louisville, KY, received the 2011 "Quality Healthcare Award" from the National Quality Forum in recognition of its efforts to "...coordinate and integrate care across the entire patient-focused experience." The Norton leaders have at least a two-decade-long commitment to quality improvement and transparency across their entire organization.

For nearly one hundred years, the Geisinger Health System has provided comprehensive care to the residents of western Pennsylvania. In 2006 its leaders launched a program called "Proven Care" based on three core elements: adherence to the highest demonstrated quality standards for care; a fixed price regardless of outcomes; and patient engagement in the decision processes throughout. Quality and innovation are cornerstones of the organization's long-term strategy, and their track record of quality improvement makes it one of the nation's strongest systems.

The Aravind Eye Care System, founded in 1976 in India, has demonstrated repeatedly that when a system is carefully designed with integrated services, it can deliver a far higher volume of eye care at a fraction of the cost with outcomes that surpass most Western systems. For example, the average number of cataract surgeries performed per hour in the Aravind system is fifteen; in the United States it is one to two. One of the higher volume eye care centers in the US is Southwestern Eye Center, where surgeons routinely operate on five to six patients per hour.

Are people who get their care in these systems healthier? We don't know. We also don't know if they are safer from preventable injuries, although these systems report significant reductions in their error rates across a number of areas. What we do know is what the clinicians and the patients say.

Like any complex enterprise, the people in these systems have a range of perspectives—they do not walk or talk in lockstep. What emerge are themes, expressed differently by different people, which describe what these organizations have accomplished. A common one, especially for physicians, is how hard this is and how different it is from the way they have always practiced. They have had to learn new ways of working together, replacing the expectations and habits of independent practice. They, as well as nurses and other clinicians, have had to learn to work in teams that may not have the hierarchies they're used to. Everyone has been forced to examine what work they do to make it better. And they have had to learn how to include the patient in the decisions about their care.

These are hard changes. The search for the right answer, the "solution," has been replaced by the best that can be found for now, and a relentless, never-ending process of improvement to make it better and better. People no longer have the security of a well-defined endpoint; they are engaged in an unending journey to learn and get better.

But the story you hear goes beyond the frustrations of leaving behind what is familiar, because the physicians and clinicians, the support staff, and leadership also describe how much better patients feel about the care they receive. They see it in the health of the system itself, the strengthening of its balance sheet, its responses to threats and challenges from the market, and its readiness for an unclear future. The journey produces tangible, measurable rewards that, for most at least, make it worthwhile in spite of the challenges. They wouldn't go back to the old way, even as they acknowledge that the changes were tough and not always pleasant.

Not everyone feels this way. There are always dissenters. Some physicians may be unable to let go of the traditional ways they've done things; they worry that letting go of their well-established habits will jeopardize the quality of the care they can provide. Or they may choose not to work in teams they do not control. They may want greater certainty, an established way to do things that doesn't change. Nurses may prefer to take orders rather than share decision-making responsibilities. Some patients may want their physicians to tell them what to do, especially when they face complex medical decisions. Throughout any organization, even ones that share the characteristics described, there are different voices, and varying reactions to the changes. The dominant theme, however, is excitement and pride. Most patients are happier with their care. Their care works for them. Working in teams is more productive and rewarding than working alone for most professionals. Shared purposes and values have created a strong community and a powerful identity.

What do patients say? What stories do they tell? The most impressive observation of all is that the stories are good and bad. Patients share their experiences with audiences inside the system in their own voices. They talk about what worked and didn't, how they felt, and what they wished had happened. The best systems don't cherry-pick the feedback to make themselves look good. They are awash with patients and their stories—good and bad—because this is how they learn to make things better. They do the usual surveys, the studies of patient satisfaction, the questionnaires, the focus groups, and the "hidden shopper" tests. They use all the tools they can muster to measure how well they serve their patients. But the most critical source is directly from the patients themselves. These organizations "marinate" in the stories. (Michael Dowling, president and CEO of North Shore-Long Island Jewish Health System, introduced me to this term.) As a result, facts and statistics have a human connection and emotional reality that forces people to listen, feel, and respond. These stories, these voices, change the conversations, which helps everyone in the organization focus on what matters to those they serve. They help identify solutions that work for them, consistent with the values and practices of the professionals and the leaders of the system. Patients ask questions that professionals and managers may hear but often don't, at least not directly: Why didn't you tell me? Why did you treat me this way? Why did you hurt me? What went wrong? Why can't you change something that doesn't work for me or for us?

Take a step back from these stories, and you hear other themes from patients too. Trust in the people of the system, in physicians and other clinicians, in the system itself, for example, because the patients know what to expect. They know what lies ahead and they hear directly from their treating clinicians when something unexpected comes up that requires a change in the plan. They understand their choices and make informed decisions about their treatment and their ongoing care consistent with their values and personal circumstances. They are partners in their care. They see that they are getting the best care possible because they look at the data with the professionals, and they participate in the decisions about their care. They feel safe. They know the clinicians know them and what is happening to them, regardless of who actually provided the care. They know, too, that they are part of a system that is obsessed with making their care as safe as possible.

They also feel this way because they are part of the evaluation of how the system and its clinicians perform for them. They have a stake in the system beyond obtaining their care from it. They participate in their own care, they join teams to evaluate and improve care, they evaluate the overall performance of the system, and they take part in strategic planning with representatives of the organization and the communities. They know their system and believe they get the best, safest care possible in it. They trust their clinicians and the system itself to act in their best interests. They recommend the care to others in the community and get care for their families there.

If these systems perform at a higher level than the rest of the systems in the country, how have they done it? What did they do to change? Many have written about organizational change. John Kotter, who has written extensively on the subject, suggests that the impetus is often a burning platform, an immediate threat to the survival of the organization. When the threat is real, it can start the ball rolling. But a transformation like the one described in this book take years, often a decade or more, to complete. You have to find a different way to sustain the effort for the long run. And you may want to use a different approach to get things started, especially if the organization is not in immediate danger.

Glenn Steele, MD, president and CEO of Geisinger Health System, worked with two cardiovascular surgeons with the desire to make things better in their service. These surgeons decided that they would treat any complication or outcome failure that occurred during their care free of charge. As far as I know, this was the first time any surgeons had guaranteed the quality of their work this way. Not surprisingly, one of the side-benefits was for the surgeons and their teams to examine everything they did to ensure that the outcomes were the very best possible. Steele built on this success to find others within Geisinger who wanted to make changes in their care. He helped them develop solutions that could benefit the institution. This is what a colleague once described as the "jujitsu" approach to change; it uses the energy someone already has to "flip" them in a direction that helps them and the organization. It is opportunistic, not strategic. It focuses on changes that are possible, that have champions, rather than on those that could be more important in the longer term. This approach is designed to build momentum. You use the results to illustrate what is possible. Once the changes start, you can move toward more strategic, targeted efforts where the payoff is greater.

Another approach is to expose your people to other organizations that have made significant improvements in their performance. The ThedaCare leadership visited a local snow-blower plant. Virginia Mason takes its leaders, including its board of directors, to Japan to train in the Toyota University. Our senior team at Kaiser Foundation Health Plan and Hospitals spent a day with the leaders at Johnson & Johnson. The goal of these visits is to see firsthand what is possible. You can't transfer the process of building cars to taking care of people. Patients aren't snowblowers. But it is instructive to see what these organizations have achieved. To get the full benefit of these visits, your team needs to explore how the lessons can apply to your own institution. You need to break through the belief that the experiences outside healthcare couldn't possibly relate to the special work we do. With well-orchestrated visits and thoughtful reflection, these direct, hands-on observations can jar us loose from this traditional thinking.

Building the new capabilities into your care delivery system is likely to be the toughest work you will undertake in your career. You are pushing against decades of tradition, reinforced by a web of expectations, laws, and regulations, and a payment system rigged against you. Change happens slowly. You must be deliberate and thoughtful in how you lead it. It is a marathon, not a sprint. The remainder of this book is an extended discussion of how to lead such a transformation. It starts with you, the leader, and how you prepare yourself to lead.

CHAPTER THREE

HOW DO YOU LEAD?

Loo Choon Yong, MD, is one of the most successful healthcare leaders I know. He combines a deep understanding of medicine with uncommon skills as a businessman. He earned a law degree while practicing medicine full-time early in his career. What began in Singapore as a two-person family practice in 1976, he has transformed into the leading group-practice-based medical care system in Southeast Asia. But a failure best showcases his true leadership capabilities.

In 2003 Dr. Loo agreed to have his neurosurgical colleagues undertake the complicated surgery to separate twenty-nine-year-old Iranian twins joined at the head. The story of the women, their difficult lives and remarkable academic achievements as law students, their search for an opportunity to live separate lives, and their willingness to undergo a dangerous surgery with a fifty-fifty chance of success, was widely reported in the international press. When they died within a short time of one another after the fifty-three hour operation that involved an international team of twenty-eight physician specialists and over one hundred support staff working in shifts, the news was broadcast around the globe.

Dr. Loo took a significant risk when he allowed his team to undertake the surgery. At the time, his hospital was only two years old. He knew he was putting its reputation and that of the Raffles Medical Group at stake. He made the choice carefully, working closely with his board and other outside advisors before deciding to go forward. He assembled an experienced, world-class team from around the globe and required them to prepare exhaustively in repeated simulation exercises prior to the surgery. He ensured that the twins had the information they needed to understand the dangers they faced, and the time and counseling to consider their choices. He was part of the team in the operating room, not as a surgeon, but to participate when the decision was made to continue forward with the operation at its most difficult stage. He wanted to be sure the wishes of the twins were represented in that choice. He was compassionate in dealing with the staff once the deaths of these popular women were announced. He made sure people had time to grieve, and had access to counseling and religious services after the unsuccessful surgery. He was transparent about the care, and, together with the physicians and nurses and others involved, he explored how they could have done things differently, how they could be better the next time. Throughout, he set a high moral bar as a sensitive clinician, a thoughtful decision-maker, a careful implementer, a flexible responder, and most of all, a compassionate human being. He stood with the team and the people who provided the care. At the same time, he never lost sight of what the impact might be on the organization he led, and he took every step possible to ensure that the care was as excellent as the caring. This is leadership.

If leadership like this is a high-stakes endeavor, transformative leadership is even more so. The rewards are great but so are the risks. What could be more satisfying than helping the people of your organization provide better, safer care to those who rely on you? Or leaving its culture and values, capabilities, quality, financial strength, and adaptability stronger than you found them? But you are exposed when you do these things, a lightning rod for criticism and anger. Physicians may blame you for their insecurities about the future. Nurses can be difficult and uncompromising. Events you don't control can disrupt your plans and provide opportunities to criticize for those who prefer the status quo or disagree with the direction you are taking.

There are other downsides too. You must expend effort and energy that are "...more than most are willing to give," as John Gardner observes in his classic work *On Leadership*. You will be lonely. You are isolated no matter how many there are around you, or how much support you receive. You will be totally absorbed. Only when you step down will you realize how completely the role dominated your life. You have to resist what John Toussaint, the former CEO of ThedaCare, described to me as the "shiny objects" that divert you from the challenges while promising exciting opportunities for personal recognition. When you seek to transform a good organization into a great one, there is little time for anything other than the day-in, day-out work to bring about the changes. And especially in healthcare you have to bridge major fault lines to do so. You have to be able to learn and grow as a result of, not in spite of, the conflicts inherent in our complex organizations.

The fissures lie just below a thin veneer of cooperation and interdependence, inhibiting collaboration and making our healthcare systems unusually difficult to lead. Physicians identify with their profession and their many specialties. Nurses do too. So do most other health professionals. Each is reinforced by laws or regulations or traditions that define who they are, how they must be prepared, and what they do. The boundaries overlap. Specialist physicians care for patients who are also the responsibility of the generalist. Nurses assume responsibilities from physicians. Nurse assistants take over work done by nurses. Every group fights for a place in the delivery system and a piece of the economic pie that feeds it. When the pie grows, tensions may be relieved, but when it is fixed or shrinking, each group fights harder. Tensions are not just economic, though. They involve control, leadership, and hegemony too. Each group is a tectonic plate that rubs against the others to create pressures that can intensify and sometimes break. When ruptures occur, the damage to the organization can be widespread and long lasting.

The fault lines are not limited to those who deliver care. A major one divides clinicians and managers, those who provide care or directly support the clinicians, and those who manage the organization. This is the San Andreas Fault of healthcare delivery, where the potential to do the most damage lies. The forces have competing imperatives and expectations. Physicians care for their patients one by one, obligated by tradition and, in one form or another, the Hippocratic Oath, to provide the best possible care to each patient, to act in the best interest of each patient, and to do no harm. Traditionally the hospitals, the nursing homes—all the places where physicians practice—were run for the physicians' benefit, a place to carry out the work for which they have trained so long. Physicians set the rules, directed the other health workers, and self-governed in accordance with medical staff bylaws they had a major role in creating. But over the past several decades, this has changed. Now there are parallel accountabilities. Physicians, and many other clinicians for that matter, have legally defined and regulated, and socially reinforced roles to play. The organization and its leaders do too. Individual physicians or the physician group (or any other clinician or support person or group that represents them) must protect individual interests and their economic viability. The organization and its leaders must protect the integrity and financial viability of the institution. While these responsibilities are often mutually reinforcing, they just as often conflict. The biggest obstacle the transformative healthcare leader faces is to bridge these fault lines when they do, to find the answers that lie hidden in the conflicts themselves.

No matter how difficult it is to change our healthcare systems, our challenges pale next to those Deng Xiaoping faced to bring China into the twentieth century. China is a country of major ethnic and social divisions, vast disparities between the wealthy and the poor, between those who live in the cities and those in the countryside, between the educated and uneducated. Deng had to bridge differences in ideologies, the rigid doctrines of Chairman Mao Tse-Tung and the market-friendly approaches of the West that had left China isolated from the rest of the world for decades.

Or look closer to home. When Abraham Lincoln assumed the presidency of the United States in 1860, the nation faced civil war. Irresolvable issues separated individuals, groups, and states. One of the best discussions of how Lincoln dealt with these challenges is the biography, *Team of Rivals* by the historian, Doris Kearns Goodwin, also the basis for the movie, *Lincoln* (2012). Goodwin focuses on the way Lincoln constructed his cabinet, interacted with a divided Congress to execute the Union's war against the Confederacy, and reached agreement to end the nation's most divisive social legacy. She describes his approach to leadership, including the characteristics that contributed to his success.

Lincoln was a student, according to Goodwin, deeply introspective, self-taught and widely read. He learned all he could about military history and strategy in order to guide the generals who led the Union forces. His views on slavery evolved throughout his life and culminated in the Emancipation Proclamation. As a result of the way he learned, he trusted his instincts and his judgments. His sense of history, his understanding of himself and the motivations of others, helped him stand apart, reach his own conclusions, and set the course he felt was best. He relied on others for advice but found the course that rang true for him. A powerful moral compass guided him through crisis after crisis, and decision after decision. Goodwin describes the long nights he sat in his study dealing with the horrors of the war, the sorrows in his personal life, and the challenges he faced in healing the nation. One is struck with the eloquence of his letters and speeches, and the profound morality and learning that shaped them.

He was also unabashedly human, unafraid to show his emotions, deeply passionate about the issues and the people he interacted with. He invited people into the White House. He took every opportunity to interact with his constituents. He received thousands of letters and responded personally to most. He wrote letters to parents who had lost their children in the war. He rarely shied from talking with the people he led. In his frequent visits to the troops on the front lines, he sat for hours listening to their concerns, telling stories, and collecting messages to send back to families. According to letters these soldiers sent home, he even cried with them.

Lincoln was also willing to stand alone. He was often at odds with those closest to him, and experienced unceasing criticism and scorn from his critics and enemies. He carried the unimaginable weight of the future of the Union on his shoulders, as well as a deep sense of responsibility to address the most profoundly divisive issue in our nation's history. He spoke often of his loneliness, but he seldom wavered in maintaining his independence or in taking positions that put him at odds with his closest advisors if he felt he was right. Yet if Goodwin's characterization is correct, he gained the respect, even friendship, of members of his cabinet and those with whom he worked most closely, despite their disagreements. He sought their advice and listened carefully to what they offered, but still reached his own conclusions and made his lonely decisions while retaining their loyalty and admiration.

Today Lincoln would be called a hands-on leader. He visited the places where work was done, asked questions, learned, worked side by side with those involved to figure out what to do and how to do it. He seemed to be everywhere. Letters home from soldiers on the front line describe his visits. Diaries kept by members of his cabinet include entry after entry about interactions with Lincoln across a range of issues and concerns. Lincoln's personal records reveal a man who reveled in the details of the work of governing.

Another trait that set Lincoln apart was his ability to find the right story or diffuse a tense situation with a funny, often ribald joke. He was a masterful storyteller, a skill he honed as a young traveling lawyer. He was not aloof or inaccessible. He could be profoundly moving, his eloquence and persuasiveness were legendary. In most settings, in spite of the dangers he faced and the war he oversaw, he used stories and real examples, laced with a humorous anecdote or a joke, to convey the points he wanted to make. He was even criticized by some for not being serious or dignified enough, for not being "presidential," but those who knew him well or had to negotiate with him found out quickly how deadly serious and focused he was.

Lincoln was a masterful politician. He defied the odds to win elections no one believed he could, outmaneuvered better-known rivals, and won battles with a Congress often dead set on thwarting him. He knew what was possible and had a refined sense of timing. He was comfortable with compromise and skilled in reaching agreements with those who opposed him. He understood what made people work, and he was sensitive to each person's desires and needs. He knew when he held the winning hand and when he didn't. He could be tough and unyielding when necessary, making unpopular decisions like firing General George B. McClellan, his first Union general. He also was able to wait when he needed to. Goodwin notes that once Lincoln decided to abolish slavery, he delayed his proclamation until he was in a strong enough position as the leader of the country to withstand the deep-seated hostility it would engender.

And finally there was his cabinet. These men really were his rivals, strong and independent, experienced, and vocal. They had run against him for office; several had been his cruel and public critics. Goodwin explores what enabled Lincoln to surround himself with men like this. One explanation is cynical: he wanted his most dangerous political foes close-by so he could watch them. President Lyndon Johnson, according to Goodwin, was fond of saying "It's better to have them inside the tent pissing out, than outside pissing in." But Goodwin argues that there was more to Lincoln's decision than this. He sought the perspectives and capabilities he needed to lead the country, without fear of strong personalities. He gave others credit when they deserved it, yet willingly shouldered responsibility even when others had made the wrong decisions. Most of all, his independence and trust in his judgment gave him the confidence to learn from others, seek their advice, and still make the decisions he needed to make. He had the integrity and intellectual strength to use the conflicts to find the best answers. Instead of shying away from disagreements or suppressing passionate debate, he used them to help him chart his course. For Lincoln, conflict was "generative," to use the word of another scholar, Diana Walsh, the former president of Wellesley College.[4]

Lincoln's character was formed during a time dominated by men, and he has been so mythologized that it is hard to separate truth from

[4] Dr. Walsh used this phrase during her speech to the participants at the Gold Lab Symposium in Boulder, CO. Walsh, Diana. (President Emerita) "Educating Our Smartest Kids to Tackle the Big Problems in Healthcare" Wellesley College, May 18, 2013

fiction. His example may not apply to our modern times or to healthcare. But certain traits of his are worth considering. To change the culture of your organization, sever some of the deepest roots of tradition, and achieve an entirely new level of care for those who seek help, you must be a student of care delivery, how patients make their decisions to seek help, and how people can be motivated to work together to create something better. You must understand how the people and the pieces can be integrated, seeking analogies from other industries, and exploring how other healthcare leaders have adapted them. You must know about motivation and timing, how to take advantage of the opportunities, the energy that you can use to change the organization. You have to be flexible, willing to change direction, choose new tactics, and rethink your assumptions as you are presented with new information and unexpected conditions. In your own style, you must be willing to show your emotions, your passions, your sadness, and your joy. You cannot shield your feelings with words that distance you from those who seek help and those who provide it. You cannot allow your position or your work to interfere with your humanity, for ultimately, this is both what drives you and connects you to those around you. You need to know enough about the issues you deal with to draw your own conclusions and make the lonely decisions that leadership requires. To do this well, you must have confidence borne of study and insight and experience, and with it the ability to seek many points of view, listen to those ideas and opinions, and shape them into decisions most likely to work. Instead of a facilitator who seeks the common ground among the competing views of others, you are a participant-leader who explores issues from many angles so the best solutions can emerge. You must know who you are to lead like this—what values and ethics define your moral character because that is the wellspring that ultimately guides you.

In the previous chapter I described the "jujitsu" approach to making changes in an organization—using the energy of others to move them in the direction you want them to take. Leadership acumen is knowing where and when the timing is right to make a particular move or take a particular step. You need this sense to lead an organization through major changes. You have to know who you can count on, what will encourage people to support a change, who the opponents are, and what they will do to block what you wish to accomplish. It is a judgment you must make every step of the way because people are affected differently at different times over different issues. It is always changing, the sand constantly shifting under your feet. You can never stop listening to your organization to determine where it has become possible to institute this experiment, or push that new approach. To use the political analogy, you must wait patiently, often working behind the scenes, until you assembles the "votes" to take another step forward. Your antennae work overtime. You use the intelligence you gather from many sources to assess the readiness to change as well as the people to watch out for. You craft solutions to win some over, or block others. You take a half step if none is possible, and wait until you can to take the full step. You take an imperfect solution over no solution, but only if doing so doesn't compromise momentum or the change effort itself.

You must draw others to your shared purpose and encourage often uncomfortable actions that can help realize that vision. You lead through stories, insights, wise and timely decisions, and the mutual trust and respect you build, always focused on those who seek our help. Patient by patient, problem by problem, opportunity by opportunity, you work hand in hand with those around you to craft solutions that meet the purpose and are consistent with the values that guide that purpose. You share the joys and the heartaches that affect us all, but assume the lonely responsibility for the most troubling, difficult decisions that must be made to create the future.

Max De Pree, the former CEO and chairman of Herman Miller Corporation, has written extensively about leadership. One work I particularly like is his second book, *Leadership Jazz: The Essential Elements of a Great Leader* (first published in 1993 and revised in 2008). De Pree suggests that leading an organization is like leading a jazz band "... because performers in organizations are often called on to make their own variations on a tune, to improvise as part of a team, to innovate in concert with others." A superb jazz leader, I would add, is usually an excellent musician who can play as well as lead; think of Duke Ellington or Tommy Dorsey. That kind of leader understands the framework: the chord changes, the timing, and the rhythms to make the music. The genius of jazz is the creativity, the breath-taking improvisation that occurs within that well-understood discipline. The leader is also comfortable disappearing into the group or the orchestra, emerging for a solo perhaps, then rejoining the group to play background for someone else, then working with the bandmates to create a sound that blends the players into one. To do this, the leader has to know each player as intimately as possible; he has to know what he wants the music to sound like; he has to know the discipline backward and forward and understand what part each musician plays to create the whole, and he must orchestrate all of them simultaneously to produce the sounds he knows are there. He also knows how to get the best, the most creative performances from his fellow musicians, how to motivate them, include them in putting the pieces and the parts together. But unlike jazz, healthcare leadership is not a single performance, and your orchestra is not an ensemble but a vast collection of individuals and teams and interests. The leader conducts day after day, year after year, in an unending search for a better and more creative care, coaxing, teaching, leading, resting, and sometimes disciplining. You conduct this complex array of people for the course of your tenure, in a steady, thoughtful, often frustratingly slow, never-ending search for the perfect performance.

CHAPTER FOUR

STARTING

When I became CEO, I wanted to establish my independence and signal that things were about to change. I made most early decisions based on the merits, but some because they were the opposite of what my predecessor had done. The circumstances of my selection complicated the situation. I was the dark-horse choice, and throughout the long transition from my predecessor, Jim Vohs, to me, speculation was rampant that some group would try to reverse the board's decision to appoint me as the new CEO.

I hadn't yet learned how to filter the rumors. The Program thrived on that sort of thing and here was an opportunity to fan the flames. Even though Jim worked hard to create a smooth transition for the Program, the fears sparked by the rumors were never far from my mind. My energies before assuming the role were directed toward getting ready and at the same time making sure the disconcerting chatter didn't become a reality. As a result, I didn't take the time to explore what people had to say to me as their new leader. I didn't fill the huge gaps in my knowledge of some regions and the potential communication channels at my disposal. And that was a mistake.

I started with an incomplete understanding of the organization, and lacked wide-ranging relationships, long-standing or recent, that could help me understand the realities that people in the organization confronted. I hadn't built the robust network to communicate informally throughout the organization. I began a few cards short of a full deck, and had to work hard to recover later when impressions had already been formed and early mistakes had slowed the transformation.

I decided when to leave my position about three years ahead of time. I wanted to make sure the board knew what my plans were, and give them ample opportunity to observe the internal candidates who might replace me. I also wanted my departure process to be as smooth as possible, with minimal speculation about the process or the timing. I also felt strongly that the sitting CEO should have no formal role in selecting his successor beyond providing the board with a slate of qualified successors from inside the organization. Our successor selection was transparent and board run. I consulted with the board from time to time at their request, but otherwise stayed out of their deliberations. Once my successor was announced, we communicated both the timing of the hand over and the process for the transition. No secrets. I made it clear that I would leave the board as soon as my successor became the chair of the board. And when George Halvorson became the CEO and chairman, I moved to a small office several floors away from the C-suite until the end of 2002 as planned. George and I have been friends and colleagues throughout his tenure, meeting informally from time to time at his request. But after 2002, I retained no formal ties to Kaiser Permanente.

How you begin your work sets the tone for your tenure. You can change direction, of course, but it is difficult because first impressions are so hard to undo. Whether or not you have actually succeeded in changing your organization will only become clear five or ten years after you've left, so preparing for your departure is as important as planning how you begin.

Planning for how you will engage your organization during those first months is an essential part of your preparation. It doesn't matter if you are new to your job or have been a member of the leadership team;

the preparation clock starts when you begin your transformation to your new leadership position. The amount of time you have for this phase depends on the circumstances of your appointment. Longer is better, up to several months if possible. But if you are part of a leadership shake-up or need to fix a damaged organization, you may have to act more quickly just to keep the organization alive.

Whatever the situation, you want to accomplish two objectives in this first stage.

Break with the Past. To build the new capacity demands a different way of leading. This is what your planned break should signal: an opportunity for the people in the organization and you to step back and take stock instead of jumping right into the fray using the same tools and assumptions that have brought you to this point. As its new leader, you want to take time to understand the organization regardless of the roles you may have had in the past. You want to guard against acting for the sake of action. You want to avoid decisions based on information and perceptions you developed before you became the leader. No matter how long you have been in the organization, you cannot expect to know enough about it yet to lead a transformation like this one. Circumstances may require you to act with incomplete information, of course. But it is quite another thing to act because you think this is what you are supposed to do, or because you succumb to the desire to establish your independence from the past by undoing decisions right away, or you make a decision—any decision—just to show that you can.

Establish the informal power that you must have to lead. As the titular leader of the organization, you have positional power. But your effectiveness depends far more on the informal power you *earn* than the formal title you *have*. Without the support and engagement of the people you lead, your transformation cannot happen. It is nearly impossible to force changes of this magnitude into a healthcare organization using positional power. There are too many ways to resist, too many divided loyalties, and too much tradition to overcome. Besides, the people who do the work of caring for patients, and the patients themselves, have the best ideas for making care better and better. You don't. Experts don't. The people who serve and who are served are the source of the energy and creativity you must have to change the organization. And for this to happen, you have to earn the right to lead them.

This is why a break at the start is so important. It gives you time to learn what the people of the organization do and what they need to do their work better. It is an opportunity to listen to them, seek out their ideas, engage with them in dreaming about what the future could be, and explore how others have made their organizations work more effectively and how to do those things in your organization. This is when you earn their trust. You listen and learn, ask questions in order to get to know the people in your organization, the patients you serve, and the people in the community. And because you are a new leader, you will hear and see things differently. You have new filters, and, when you ask, people will tell you things they want you to hear as their new leader. It is their opportunity to help you understand who they are, what they understand about the organization and its future, and what they need to get there.

This moment of openness is ephemeral; it disappears quickly. Every opinion you express and decision you make closes a door somewhere in the organization as the people form their views of you, what you stand for, what you will accept or focus on, and what you won't. It's inevitable. You want to keep alive your opportunity to learn and develop your informal power base as long as you can. Ideally, you'd close no doors, but that isn't realistic. You are the leader. You stand for certain things; you want to accomplish certain goals, and lead the organization in a particular direction. Every choice you make creates ripples. But you want to extend this special time for as long as you can in order to build the relationships you need.

Informal power depends on how well you make sense of what is happening in and around the organization, as well as how effectively you establish relationships at multiple levels both inside the organization and out. Your words and actions, and ultimately the decisions you make, all contribute to the picture that people form about you. And this picture determines whether or not they are willing to join you, give you the benefit of their energy and creativity. This is the informal power you seek: the ability to convince people to join you in this long journey and to earn their trust and confidence so that the entire organization can benefit from their energy, ideas, and commitment to a different future.

Your informal power also is most powerfully determined by the values you share with those around you. Before they agree to join you, they must trust that you believe as they do about the purpose of the organization, about what you can do together, and the way you do it. This period early in your tenure is when your messages are clearest, before the noise of daily demands and decisions drowns out what you hope to convey. How you spend your time and how you act in these early months is your best opportunity to demonstrate the core importance of superior quality, as well as three key values for the transition ahead: (1) constant learning; (2) all voices matter; and (3) there is no we-they, you are in this together. People will notice because this is when they are most open to understanding who you are and what you represent.

You may be able to convey these messages through carefully selected actions. When Paul O'Neill became CEO of Alcoa Aluminum, he established credibility with the employees through a series of early actions and decisions to create a safe workplace in an industry notable for injuries and even deaths. More likely, you will do it by spending time with the people who practice and work in the organization, and from the people you serve.

The informal power you need requires a foundation of shared values with those who serve and are served by your organization; relationships based on a shared understanding of what is possible and what stands in the way; and stories and insights that make sense of what occurs today and can be done tomorrow. The breathing space in the first few months is designed to help you accomplish these objectives. Described below are several guidelines for how to make this happen.

- **Allocate sufficient time.** This is your top priority. You must carve out time every day to spend listening and learning. During the first months, you will want to spend up to 75 percent of your time doing this. Later you will have to decrease the time, perhaps to 50 percent or even one third of your time, due to the press of other business. Whatever number you select, be religious about making sure it happens. Block it out on your calendar. Plan how you will use the time. Make the arrangements so it is hard to procrastinate, and difficult for other demands to impinge on the time. Assign someone in your office to manage this for you.

- **Identify the targets.** Identify the people you want to meet and where you want to meet them. Decide ahead of time whether or not these interactions will be one-on-one meetings, small groups, or in larger gatherings. You will want to use all three, though the individual and small group discussions are likely to be the richest. Balance your inside and outside focus so you spend equal time with the people who serve and those who are served. Talk with representatives from the community too. The person who manages your calendar can help you keep track of where you go and whom you see.

- **Define your process in advance.** You want to define a general process as well as a specific approach to each interaction. As a general rule, you want to speak less than 50 percent of the time, and ideally shoot for talking less than 25 percent of the time. You do this by asking questions rather than speaking or offering opinions. Try to save your remarks for the end, and limit them to answering questions that the individual or people in the group might have. If you do feel the need to convey the importance of the core values—superior quality, learning, all voices matter, we're in this together—do it briefly and simply, then let your actions speak by seeking information, learning all you can, listening carefully to each person who speaks, thanking each person personally for their ideas, and refraining from judgments as much as possible. This is not the time to discuss strategy or tactics, nor is it yet the time to lay out your vision for the future except in the broadest terms. Your objective is to learn from others, and to hear what they have to say.

Plan each interaction in advance to be sure you are focused on the particular issues that person or that part of the organization may have. You want to ask good questions and establish the relationships built on your understanding and interest in their work and their lives. The person you've assigned to manage your calendar may be able to pull together the background information you will need. Before you go into any interaction, identify specific issues you'd like to explore and questions you want to ask. Remind yourself about the talk-listen ratio and what your purpose is.

At the end of each day it is a good idea to make brief notes about what you've learned and what insights you have gained. You also want to send a thank you to each person: a brief handwritten note, an e-mail, or, depending on the situation, something even more personal like a bouquet of flowers (you may have learned, for example, about the birth of a child, a celebration of some sort, or even an illness or death; any one of those things deserves a personal response from you). Make sure you allocate the time for this too. It doesn't need to take long, not more than thirty minutes or so most days.

- **Delay decisions and actions as long as you can (except the ones that communicate your core values).** You will be under intense pressure to make decisions in your new role. You want to establish your credibility as the leader and, traditionally, the way we do this in our action-oriented society is to do things, act, decide. I urge you to remember what a surgeon advised us as young medical students, "For heaven's sake, don't do anything. Observe carefully, observe again, and then you might be ready to act." You only get one shot at taking time like this to learn about the organization from the people who work there and are cared for there. Take full advantage of it. Don't confuse the messages you will want to convey throughout your tenure by making premature or hasty decisions, however pressured you may feel. Organizational inertia will push things ahead; you don't have to reinforce it. Critical decisions will get made. Your biggest concern is to build your informal power, the power that enables you to lead over the long term. Short-term decisions are less important in the beginning. Delegate them to others; let them happen if they don't send the wrong messages about who you are and what you hope for. Otherwise don't make them; avoid them; delay them as long as you can.

- **Use all tools to communicate.** The language of leadership includes what you say, what you do, and how you act. You communicate through these mediums, recognizing that you are both a person who leads and the symbol of the leader. In this early period, you want to be mindful of the fact that your actions and statements have an especially powerful impact on the organization. This is the time when people watch you most closely, reading the tea leaves to see what is important to you, determining where they fit in this new scheme of things. It is a period of testing and formation. Your words matter, you have to choose them with care. How you spend your time, where you spend it, and with whom, sends even louder signals throughout the organization. And finally, the questions you ask, the way you listen and respond, the way you follow up with thank-you notes and recognition add to the picture that people create.

The day you begin you should start to prepare a well-thought-out succession plan for you and your leadership team. It takes time to develop the next generation of leaders, to prepare them to continue the organization's journey toward superior care. Typically, however, these plans do not include a specific timetable. You may have a notion of how long you expect to be in your job, but, if you are like most of us, you won't think about it very much until the time to depart gets close. I urge you to approach this differently. Right from the start, you should be clear with yourself how long you expect to be in your role. Be as specific as you can. You may or may not share it with your board of directors, but you certainly want an understanding with yourself.

On the day Bill George signed his contract to begin as CEO and chairman of Medtronic, he submitted his letter of resignation for a date ten years in the future. His board had the right to terminate him before that, but he was unwilling to stay longer. He believed that CEO effectiveness diminishes after ten years, and that every organization needs new leadership to recharge and refocus. I wasn't convinced when he shared this opinion with me. But not long after that conversation, and for different reasons, I informed my board that I planned to leave in three years. Before that we had worked on succession planning, and done the "hit by the bus" exercise almost every year to agree on who would take on the leadership role in the event of unexpected death or disability. Once I shared the specific timetable for my departure, though, I realized that Bill George was right. I wish I had done it earlier. There are four reasons why:

It changes your relationship with the organization. Leadership is seductive. You can easily fall into the trap of believing that the organization cannot survive without you. The reverse may be true too; you may have difficulty imagining how you can live after you step aside. An important perspective is lost when this happens, when you act as though you are indispensable to the organization or vice versa. Like it or not, you are in your role for a finite amount of time. Someone probably had the job before you did; others will follow. You expect the organization will outlive you. When you set a date for your departure, you remind yourself that you are part of this cycle. Establishing at the outset when you plan to leave means that you know you will, that you are a temporary resident in the office. You are more likely to keep one foot solidly inside the organization and another outside, helping you maintain your perspective, see the organization more objectively, and not conflate the pressures you may feel as leader with those the organization must address to be successful.

It changes the way you set priorities. Setting a date for your departure as CEO is like deciding on a date for a big trip. Only when you know when you are leaving do you focus on what you have to do to prepare. Priorities shift, different demands move ahead in the queue because you know how long you have to work on your agenda. This is especially critical when you want to make major changes. You can't afford to be distracted by other priorities or let important milestones slip. You can't lose focus. When you are ambiguous about the amount of time you have ahead of you, you can procrastinate, let other demands move to the front of the queue, and put off the hard stuff until later. Knowing when you will leave sharpens your attention to what you need to do before you go.

It changes your willingness to deal with conflicts and controversies. As we've already discussed, the biggest obstacle to changing your course is the traditional culture. There is no way to lead an organization on the journey like this one without conflict and controversy. In my experience, we often find ourselves trying to maintain equilibrium in the organization, "keeping the peace" on the one hand, and driving forward with the changes on the other. We put off the hard decisions, or we soften them because we believe we can revisit them later. It seems to be human nature to do this when we believe we have more time. Most of us don't like conflict. We don't like to make people angry or upset. We prefer to fudge, to soften, and will keep doing so as long as we can.

Your views shift when you know how long you expect to be in the job. You become more strategic, stronger even. You decide which tough decisions you will take on, and in which order. You are less concerned with being liked and getting along, and more with doing the important things. You are less likely to avoid controversy and conflict. You may not enjoy it more, but you are more likely to deal with the really difficult decisions that are part of this transformation.

It changes the amount of attention you give to hardwiring the changes so they endure after you leave. The last thing you want is for the organization to "snap back" to the old way of doing things when you leave. Organizations tend to return to their original shape unless critical changes are hardwired, unless the organization is rebuilt to reinforce the new culture and reject the old one. The focus of this book is really about those changes and the hardwiring required to make them happen. When you know that your part in the race will not continue indefinitely, you are less likely to neglect the work of ensuring that every important change becomes part of the ongoing culture. A thoughtful leader doesn't need this reminder, but I've found that setting a date certain for leaving sharpens your focus significantly.

CHAPTER FIVE

OBSTACLES AND TRAPS

"Loss aversion is a powerful conservative force that

favors minimal changes from the status quo in the lives

of both institutions and individuals."

— **Daniel Kahneman** in *Thinking, Fast and Slow*

OBSTACLES

You cannot anticipate all the obstacles you will encounter as you move forward in your journey. Most you can manage on the fly, though some will surprise you and may knock you off course if you don't respond effectively. Four obstacles in particular represent major challenges to your change efforts and require planning in advance to minimize their effects. Most difficult by far is the strong resistance you will get from those rooted in the traditional culture of twentieth century medical care. This entire book focuses on how to deal with that resistance. In this chapter I consider three additional concerns. The financial incentives in the current system often penalize you for doing what is right for patients. Legal and regulatory requirements impede care integration and create unwanted legal exposure as well. Finally, there are "bandwidth" limits within your organization that dictate the pace at which you can make the desired changes.

Financial

You don't get paid to commit financial suicide. Many things that would benefit our patients cause financial harm to the institution. This is especially true when it comes to improving care. Examples abound. You can shorten lengths of stays in the hospital by simplifying the admissions procedures, improving coordination among specialists, speeding the diagnostic tests, and reducing post-operative recovery time. You can reduce the prevalence of hospital-acquired infections and the problems associated with errors in drug administration. The result is better, faster, safer, and less costly care for the patient, but possibly less revenues for your institution too. You may be able to backfill, to put another patient in the now-available bed, so the net result could be more, not less revenue per bed. On the other hand, you might find that demand for hospitalization overall goes down, and as a result, your income per bed is reduced. Another example is when you build a comprehensive primary care capability that includes prevention and early screening for the community. Patients are able to identify and treat their illnesses earlier in the course of the disease, and experience lower morbidity and mortality as a result—a positive outcome for them. But the rate of hospitalization for the acute manifestations of these conditions goes down too. Unless you can backfill with other patients, your overall revenues suffer. To be fair, if you can reduce overall hospitalization but still capture the revenues associated with the alternative intervention, you may be able to reduce demand for hospital beds. This can delay or avoid the capital-intensive decision to build more beds, usually a good thing, as an investment like this requires substantial capital, the approval and construction process is lengthy, the payback period is often quite long, and the opportunity costs are significant.

So how can you move forward in the face of an obstacle like this, one so serious and potentially career-shortening? I can't answer the question for you specifically because each situation is unique. But I can offer some suggestions. At the outset it is important to remember that changing your organization is a slow process, accomplished in increments rather than all at once. This is particularly important when you address the financial obstacles. You need to be strategic and clever, looking for opportunities to learn, build momentum, and generate more, not less revenues whenever you can. So how do you do this? Below are several ideas. They are not mutually exclusive, and they should be tailored to your circumstances.

- **To begin.** If you don't start with an organization in the black, it is irresponsible to build major new capabilities until you are. There is an exception. If you are losing money and believe the cause relates to poor care, you may want to begin the changes immediately. On the other hand, if you believe it is possible to get back into the black with some adjustments only, this is your first priority. Once you are in the black, you can start your major change process.

- **Invest up front.** Right from the start, you have to commit financial resources to educate your board, your leadership team, and key leaders in the organization about what you want to accomplish for patients. This doesn't have to be a large expense. If you take a team to visit a nearby company that uses the Lean production management approach, you will have only the expense of the transportation and the downtime for the team itself. If you go further afield, like Virginia Mason has done by sending team after team to Japan, the expenses are far higher. You may want to introduce the team to the model and methods you've chosen by bringing in an outside consultant/educator. Whatever approach you choose, you do not want to be penny-wise and pound-foolish. You should budget generously, including paying physician leaders for their loss of income for time away from their clinics or other income-producing activities. Including this at the outset instead of waiting for it to surface later, sends a strong signal that you are serious and prepared to put your money where your mouth is from the start.

- **Least damaging pilot(s).** It can be valuable to identify places where learning to deliver better care will cause the least damage financially, and perhaps, even benefit the organization if the chips fall the right way. This is usually in a relatively small area of operations. It should be an area that matters to patients and demonstrates to others in the organization the positive impact of the changes. Some of the obvious places where this approach has been used successfully are throughput and safety improvements in pre-op and post-op care, coordination improvements in ICU and CCU care, improved contact to definitive treatment processes related to stroke and myocardial infarction, etc. In each case the impact on the patient can be significant, even life-saving, while the negative impact on revenues is either small or nonexistent. In instances where the institution is already paid in some form of bundled payment, as noted in the next suggestion, the net impact may actually be to improve revenue realization.

- **Bundled payment, contract payment opportunities, etc.** When you are paid on some sort of bundled payment basis, you are rewarded for maximizing efficiency and quality. If, in addition, there is a performance premium for good outcomes, or a penalty for bad ones, the incentives to improve quality are even greater. You want to identify the conditions where a bundled payment exists or could exist through contracts with payers or employers. It is in these areas that improvements in care can produce financial benefits to the institution. It's a win all the way around. Insurers especially are beginning to experiment with different forms of bundled or contract payments. As you gain experience and demonstrate the impacts on patient outcomes and overall costs of care in your institution, you have a strong argument for seeking further bundled or contract payment solutions. In the absence of full capitation for a defined population, this incremental approach moves you along the path to the best care possible while benefiting you financially along the way.

The regulations for accountable care organizations provide flexibility in how you move ahead too, offering different levels of commitment and risk, and alternative payment schemes. These will change with time, as will the opportunities that exist with private payers. You want your financial team to be well versed in these options and on top of the rapidly changing reimbursement environment as well. By maintaining flexibility and continuing to learn by prudent experiments, you can find a path through the financial obstacles. It makes no sense to assume that because you have always worked with fee-for-service based reimbursements, there is no alternative. You have plenty of choices.

- **Special arrangements with employers.** Another approach is to work with local employers to develop pilots and programs that serve their employees and address their financial needs. Several healthcare organizations have done this successfully. Here the intent is to identify areas of need and fashion solutions that speed the care process and accelerate the return to productive work. You benefit in several ways. You provide better care, which enhances your morale and reputation; you build a stronger partnership with your customers; and you increase the demand for these solutions from other employers and patients who hadn't previously used your services. These are momentum enhancers. The success of working with an employer-as-partner can spur other experiments; it gets easier with each experience to build these collaborative efforts that are so essential to delivering the best care possible.

- **Innovation funds.** You should create a fund for innovation and improvement (for more details, see chapter sixteen). Given the pace of change in healthcare, investing in delivery innovations is likely to be a more rewarding expenditure than the purchase of yet another technology or the expansion in bed capacity. Compared to other industries, healthcare delivery systems have been poor at building their innovation engines. Every dollar, it seems, is earmarked to fund day-to-day operations. Investing in something amorphous, possibly even frivolous, like innovation seems a waste. Except that innovation does not have to be poorly defined or an expensive indulgence. Successful companies are disciplined in the way they innovate, planning carefully and holding themselves accountable to deliver returns for their investments in this kind of research and development. To change your course, you undertake what in effect is a major innovation effort. You have to discover what works and how to create and build momentum in your institution. An investment in innovation is a part of this. I cannot suggest a specific target; it depends on where you are as an organization. The ranges are large across other industries: from a low of 2 to 3 percent of gross revenues to upwards of 20 to 30 percent in industries that depend on innovation and discovery for their future success. Healthcare delivery falls toward the lower end, in my view, as margins are already compressed. Starting with a 3 to 5 percent allocation, you can fund what you need to, especially if you couple this level of investment with the other suggestions already mentioned.

- **Foundation or community support.** It is sometimes possible to obtain funding from local foundations or community groups to address a significant community health problem. An example of this approach is found at Mt. Sinai Hospital in Chicago, where, through their Urban Health Institute, the hospital leaders have joined with community leaders to obtain foundation support for attacking problems in obesity, diabetes, and childhood asthma.

Whichever approach works for your system, you must always move the changes forward. You do it by providing a learning and skill development opportunity for members of the workforce, by showcasing how these efforts improve the health of patients, by facilitating the development of effective partnerships between providers and patients, and between the institution, the employers, and the members of the communities you serve. You have to do this incrementally—it is simply too big to do otherwise. You must be thoughtful and systematic as you move forward with the changes so you can work through the financial barriers that you will encounter. Careful planning, including working with your board and leadership team to create the funding for the early education and innovations, will help you avoid damage to your bottom line that jeopardizes the financial health of your institution.

Legal and Regulatory

Health law is complex and in flux, especially since the Supreme Court decision about the Patient Protection and Affordable Care Act (the so-called ACA). You are certain to encounter legal and regulatory conflicts as you change your organization. It is imperative, therefore, to engage expert legal advice from a firm that specializes in health law and regulatory matters. A generalist is unlikely to have the depth or resources to do this well enough for your needs. You also want more than one-off legal advice; you need an ongoing relationship with a firm that can help you craft solutions to the legal and regulatory obstacles you will certainly encounter as you move forward. At some point you may even want to hire a full-time legal advisor to be part of your leadership team, serve as your counselor, and bridge with the legal community as specific issues arise. Expect to pay for these services. They are not cheap. But you risk damaging the organization or slowing or halting the transformation without them.

Bandwidth

The final obstacle is not having the right people and resources to do the job. People who are already committed are somehow able to stretch even more, at least for a while. They will add to their already full workloads and take on additional responsibilities. It is possible to get more from existing resources until the limits are reached. Then the bottom starts to fall out. Agreed-to priorities go unaddressed. Work priorities become jumbled. Frustration grows. Mistakes are made. It is a common problem. It can take another form too. Because people in healthcare are smart and well educated, there is often a perception that what others do isn't as difficult, or can be learned. This is especially true with physicians. You may find that people in the organization prefer to take on the new work themselves rather than hiring additional outside resources with the requisite expertise. This tendency to undershoot can cripple your transformation effort.

You can avoid this in two ways. First, you have to educate yourself and be sure the other leaders in the organization have learned how successful organizations have built the bandwidth needed to succeed. Second, you have to educate your board and leadership team about why and how much you plan to invest to drive the changes you are instituting. You must invest in training for your people, and to bring more robust information technologies into the organization. You must invest to develop data, analyze results, create improvements, implement and then assess them again in that continuous cycle. You invest to develop a cadre of people with the expertise needed to help the people of the organization do this work. You invest to get better. You can get there on the cheap for a while. But at some point you'll reach your limits and more help will be required. That point comes sooner than you expect. If you aren't prepared, you will lose valuable time and momentum, and worse yet, create a backlash in the organization that solidifies resistance.

TRAPS

Nobody's perfect. You will fall into many traps on your journey. The most significant is the delusion that there is a silver bullet for transforming your organization, or perhaps, a small collection of things that will trigger the massive changes needed. I hope you won't fall into this trap, that you don't ignore the approaches I suggest in this book. Unfortunately there is no simple answer. It doesn't work that way. You need to use every tool, small and large, to establish the capabilities you seek. Five other traps can cause you no end of headaches:

The Bubble-Boy Trap

The original "bubble boy" lacked the immune system to protect himself and was forced to live in a germ-free bubble until his death at age twelve. Leaders construct their own bubbles. They surround themselves with trusted people, deal with the pressing issues, and triage out the less relevant and less agreeable. No leader can survive without doing some of this; but it is a trap.

It is a trap because it becomes an echo chamber; you begin to hear yourself talking through those around you. You know each other so well, know the expectations so clearly, that you reinforce the assumptions and approaches you share. You listen to the same sources and interpret them the same way. You erect barriers to keep people away who disagree or aren't part of your inner circle. As you become increasingly comfortable in your role and familiar with the organization, you make assumptions about what is happening and how information should be weighed. You "filter" to manage incessant demands and never-ending challenges, and in the process create the trap that isolates you from what is really going on.

You have to escape this bubble if you want unvarnished insights into what is happening in your organization. You have to seek out dissidents, talk with the naysayers, and listen to the critics. You need lines of communication that extend your reach beyond those who share your bubble. You have to schedule time in the organization to listen and to learn, and to participate in solving problems with those affected by them. You have to wander through the organization to expose yourself to what happens there each day, to what works and what doesn't, to who helps and who doesn't. You need to see your people and hear them for yourself.

The same with patients. You must sit with them, visit them in their homes, and spend time with those who have been harmed or disappointed by what you provided them. You need to talk with people who are angry, just as you welcome the chance to listen to those who are grateful. You must deliberately weaken the protective power of your bubble. Your senior team can help if it includes people with distinct views and rich networks, and if you have created a sense of safety and a commitment to learning that encourages them to share unpleasant news, constructive criticism, unwelcome problems, and different ideas. However you do it, you must escape the way it limits what you know and see, hear, and feel.

The "Shiny Objects" Trap

A consultant left the firm where he'd worked for more than a decade to become CEO of a large international company. It was a dream job that, by all accounts, he performed exceptionally. Yet after two years, he returned to his former role. His reason? Part of the job was to give the same message time after time, day after day, employee group after employee group. He hated the repetition, the day-to-day slog. He preferred the stimulation of new ideas and different challenges, and was wise enough to realize that if he gave in to these preferences, it would harm his company. Leadership inconsistency is a curse. It can throw the organization into a tailspin and bring good work to a halt. It can de-motivate the motivated, and provide fuel to the naysayers.

Inconsistency like this takes many forms. It can be as simple as messages that don't connect or decisions without context. It can be a failure to explain how a change of tactics is not a change in basic strategy. It can be actions that are inconsistent with rhetoric, or confusion seeded by actions that appear to conflict. And it can be the "shiny objects" of leadership that divert a leader's attention to the next important matter.

Whatever the cause, it is yet another trap. You cannot expect to be perfectly consistent throughout your tenure. Few people can. But you must try. You have to try to do the same things again and again, give the same message over and over long after you are bored to tears doing so. Like Tony Bennett. Everywhere he performs he is asked to sing "I Left My Heart in San Francisco." How many thousands of times has he sung those words? Yet he performs it each time like the first time, the words fresh, the melody his own. His consistency is legendary. You have to be like Tony Bennett. People need that consistency; carrying out a successful transformation demands it.

To do this you need to protect yourself from the distractions that bedevil every leader. You have to identify the few critical priorities that will make or break your efforts to transform the organization, then manage your calendar to ensure that these are where you focus most of your time. Some suggest a leader should spend at least 70 percent of her time on these priorities. I think it should be higher when you seek to build the organizational capacity to deliver the best care possible—probably closer to 80 to 90 percent of your available time. And you should probably have just two to three priorities at any one given time. That's all you can do well and probably the limit for an organization too. Otherwise the priorities become confused or ignored. You need to do a regular time-use audit to see whether or not you have allowed "shiny object creep" to occur. Like a vigorously growing bush, you have to regularly prune your commitments and your schedule. You have to get rid of the lower priorities, the ones that add no value to your goal. You have to be ruthless. Either something contributes directly to your long-term objectives, or it is an organizational maintenance responsibility that only you can discharge. Anything else is a shiny object; get rid of it. And you have to do this regularly because in spite of your best efforts, those distractions, those shiny objects, find their way onto your calendar and sow the seeds of inconsistency that weaken your ability to lead.

The Hubris Trap

As a leader, you inevitably meet people who kiss up to you, tell you how good you are, and point out the things you've done well. You may get praise for something you've done, or for your leadership, or receive outside recognition for improvements and even the changes you've made. It's hard to resist. After all, who doesn't like praise? But watch out! When you start to believe what people say about you, you have fallen into the hubris trap. Unchecked, you develop a misplaced confidence in your own views, insights, and skills. You believe your own press, and this poses a real danger.

It manifests itself in many ways. You stop listening as much, spend more time talking, and develop an unhealthy attachment to your own ideas. The humility you may have started with gives way to a belief that you understand what others do not and have answers that no one else can provide. You dismiss dissenting opinions, stop considering ideas that differ from your own, defend your solutions, and fight those who criticize.

Being a leader is seductive and hubris is the consequence. It develops from the leader's "bubble" mentioned earlier, and results from listening only to people who tell you that you are right. That's what happened to the leaders at Enron Corporation. They were convinced that they had the answers and no one else did. They believed they knew more than anyone else, that they were smarter than the others. And they ignored signals that didn't fit their views until their house of cards crashed down around them.

We've all fallen into that trap. There's no way to avoid it. There are, however, simple ways to guard against getting so far into the trap that you cannot escape. In successful venture capital and private equity firms, investors guard against misplaced confidence through a disciplined diligence process to encourage dissent before making most investment decisions. You can do the same thing. You can ask a large number of people who know about the subject what they think about a particular issue or opportunity. Make diligence like this an integral part of your decision process on any issue of consequence. Resist the temptation to tell others what you think too soon. If you're talking more than 50 percent of the time, you're selling, not listening. Make yourself ask questions. In fact, lay out the questions ahead of time so that you have a good idea of what you need to know or confirm in order to make a decision. You have to challenge yourself to be sure you don't fall into the hubris trap. It's especially easy to start to believe one's own way of thinking, one's own conclusions, and to sidestep the discipline that can help you avoid doing so. You need to be disciplined to protect yourself from the natural tendencies most of us have.

Of course, if you have successfully built a culture of improvement and innovation, you will have surrounded yourself with people who ask why and how, who challenge the traditional ways of caring for patients and doing things, who challenge each other and you. This is the strongest antidote of all.

The "Kumbaya" Trap

How wonderful it would be if we could solve every problem, deal with every conflict, create each element of our strategy, and face every challenge by climbing into a communal hot tub, linking arms, and singing "Kumbaya"? It is so much easier if we get along, especially when the everyday work of healthcare is so intensely emotional. Surrounded by the scared, the sick, and the dying, healthcare professionals must rely on each other. Why is it not best to find a solution that satisfies us all? Most of the time it is. That's why "Kumbaya" decision-making is so common in our institutions. But it doesn't always work, and it can even make things worse. It, too, is a trap if it's the only way you do things.

Sometimes it is an individual matter; a physician throws her weight (and instruments) around like an overgrown child or a high-revenue-producing physician refuses to go along with the will of the medical group. Sometimes it is one faction or another within the organization that refuses to budge. Sometimes it is a tough decision that will produce pain for everyone but is in the best interest of the organization in the long run. In circumstances like these, the "Kumbaya" approach doesn't work; it is simply not robust enough to resolve the issue no matter how long you sit in the tub and sing together. You have to use different approaches because you cannot let the stalemate stop the progress you need to make as an organization; you may have to be unilateral, you may have to draw a line in the sand to force the issue, or you may have to take the heat. You can count on being criticized, and generating ill will. It isn't comfortable. However, if you plan well and ensure that you have the right support, you can escape the trap of the "Kumbaya" mode without jeopardizing your job or your institution.

The "I'm Owed" Trap

This may be the most insidious and damaging trap of all. You begin your leadership tenure feeling fortunate, excited, challenged, and perhaps even a bit overwhelmed. You may start with the view that you are a servant to the organization, the people of the organization, and, most importantly, the patients themselves. But if you aren't watchful, that equation can shift. You can begin to feel that the organization owes you respect, rewards, power, and prestige for the work you do for it. The shift is subtle. For example, instead of an open discussion about compensation with the board of directors, you believe the organization owes you a certain package for the work you do, and you won't budge from that demand regardless of other realities that the organization must address. Or you may want the benefits a leader has negotiated in another organization, even though they set you apart from others in your institution.

However it manifests, the underlying danger is the same: you believe you are entitled to something because of your role, your success, or your importance (hubris again). Like the other common traps, this is a sign that you have lost sight of why you do what you do and who you do it for. It is time to reassess your priorities and reestablish your connection with your moral "true north." You have to step away, gain perspective, and reboot, because if you don't, your effectiveness as a leader will plummet. You cannot motivate others to make the sacrifices they need to as a team when you expect special treatment from the organization. And it is difficult to lead the organization when you've built a special set of compensation and benefits for yourself or your senior leadership team that provides disproportionate rewards compared to the rest of the organization.

That said, it is important to have fair, open, and reasonable discussions about your relationship to the institution: how you are paid, what benefits you will receive, what you are expected to accomplish, and how you will be rewarded. Like everyone in the organization, you want to be treated fairly by those who employ you. Your responsibility in these negotiations is to be fair too. Let's be realistic. Concerns about status and pay will never go away. But you should be able to look every person in the organization in the eye and describe how you are treated, what you receive, how you are paid, and why this is appropriate. When you start to believe that you deserve things others don't, that the organization owes you, and that you are entitled to it, it becomes a real stretch to justify this to others whose support and creativity you must rely on.

These are the common and dangerous traps of leadership. To avoid them you have to know the early warning signs that alert you to the trouble ahead. No one has perfect insight though. You need help from trusted colleagues, friends, and your family. They are the mirrors that help you see yourself as others do. They enable you to step away from yourself far enough to regain your perspectives. And it is critically important that you do. Traps like these can damage, and even destroy your effectiveness as a leader. By knowing what to watch for, you have a good chance of avoiding them entirely or catching them early enough to escape their more dangerous consequences.

CHAPTER SIX

YOUR HEALTH

As we moved from Santiago, Chile, to Seattle, Portland, Denver, and then to the Bay Area during my career, my wife and I agreed that we would pay more to buy homes relatively close to work so I would waste less time commuting. This meant we could better balance professional and personal responsibilities, and both be involved in raising our children. I was able to get home more easily for family dinners, help our children with schoolwork, coach their teams, and attend their school events. It also meant I didn't extend the workday or exhaust myself driving to and from the office. I could also leave for work a little later in the morning, with more time to exercise and help out at home. And if some emergency arose at school with one of the children, it was easier to take care of it or go to the school to find out what had happened. This choice did more to protect our family, our relationship, and our health than any other I can recall.

Most of us have spent years pushing ourselves one step further, adding one more task, and taking on one more problem. We "blivet," or try to pound seventy-five pounds of horse manure into a fifty-pound bag, as they said in the military back in World War II. So we are chronically tired, don't stay in shape, and lose perspective. Things work out for us most of the time, but it is devastating when they don't. We waste time, lose momentum, make unnecessary mistakes, and jeopardize our leadership or even the organization itself. And worst of all our personal lives can fall apart.

I suspect that you already know how to maintain some balance in your life; you must to have gotten as far as you have. As a leader, though, the challenges you face increase dramatically, especially if you are making significant changes in the organization. *You* are where "the buck stops." You are responsible for what happens with every patient and with your organization. You answer to multiple stakeholders, deal with the priorities and issues, the crises and threats that occur every day, and still must maintain focus on the myriad changes required to change the course of the organization. What has worked in the past may not work as you go forward; you will probably need a better plan.

That plan should address the key areas of vulnerability you will face as a leader. Stress is high and chronic, so you should plan for how you will deal with it. Physical stamina is necessary to maintain the long hours required over the years you will be in your job. Mental stamina is important too; as a leader you have to be "on" when you are in public and attending meetings. Emotional strength is essential; you must have the ability to maintain your steadiness and poise, your sense of humor, and your perspective through the inevitable ups and downs. These aren't trivial issues. You cannot expect to meet these demands by doing an occasional turn in the gym, or a long weekend away a couple of times a year. You must establish the habits, actions, and commitments that help you maintain your health and energy for the long term. There is no formula; each of us will do it differently. Nonetheless, you might consider the following:

Exercise

The health benefits of regular exercise are well established. The private time involved in regular exercise, coupled with the workout itself, can be restorative. A routine works best, something that doesn't require much thinking or preparation. Whether your time is when you roll out of bed, come home from the office, or take a break during the day, just put on the shoes, and go for whatever time you've programmed for this. Every day. It helps to find a form of exercise that lets the mind go free.

Diet

This is tough. There are so many meetings—many of which begin or end the day—that it can be difficult to stick to a healthy eating pattern. You grab food on the go, often whatever is in front of you at a particular meeting. Your days are unpredictable, so it is often hard to know when you will be able to eat, let alone where or what you'll order. Yet like regular exercise, a good diet is essential. The more you can routinize the meal process—time, quantity, nutrients, etc.—the safer you will be. Planning ahead is crucial. Habits and routines help. Even scheduling half an hour for quiet time at lunch to eat, put your feet up, think about the day, or a problem can be helpful. The point is, you need to design how, where, and what you will eat to maintain your energy and health in the face of the leadership challenges.

Sleep

I haven't found anything that is particularly useful to deal with lack of sleep—often described as the most common health problem in the US. Some people are lucky. They sleep eight hours no matter what. Some can get by without much sleep. Most of us don't work this way so it is essential to build some kind of routine to help out. Each of us has to find our own pattern. Whatever it is, the importance of sleep cannot be overstated. You need the time to recharge and restore yourself. You need the energy and ability to discipline yourself during the day, the focus and intensity required to drive an organization ahead. You can't do it if you're always tired, at least not for very long. One thing to think about is to steep yourself in the science of sleep (as well as diet and exercise) so you can explore various ways to get the sleep you need.

Alone Time

Between the demands of the job and your family, it can be hard to find time to be alone, to reflect and think. It's often one of the first things to go. It doesn't take much time each day or each week, though. It isn't about immersing yourself in some other demanding activity. It's about time to reflect, relax, restore yourself, and find your true north again. We all need this time. Some do it through meditation or religious observance. Some do it when they walk or run. Some garden or listen to music or read a good book. This kind of time is probably best scheduled on a regular, weekly, if not daily, basis. There's value as well, in scheduling activities that enable you to leave the office behind for longer periods of time: special getaway weekends, pursuit of hobbies, longer holidays, for instance. Again, the intent is to provide breathing space. It's a chance to forget for a while, and to take the pressure off.

Family Time

It is sad to see a successful, hard-working executive find out too late that her children are in trouble because of behavioral problems, drugs, or poor grades; or that her marriage is destroyed because she has given more to her work than to her family. Problems like these can sneak up on you. You think you make adjustments along the way; you accommodate the urgent demands from your children or take a special vacation with your spouse, but if work takes most of your energy, the safe harbor of your family, the well-being of your children, and the depth and stability of your relationship with your spouse can slowly disintegrate.

There's no need for this to happen. You *can* decide how you plan to balance the competing demands. Are weekends sacrosanct? Will you be home most nights for dinner? Will you coach your children's teams during the year? Will you pay more for a home to live closer to work? How often will you get away with your spouse during the week? For special vacations? How about as a family? What are your "rules" about bringing work home? Do you do that after the kids go to bed? For how long? You get the idea. The plan isn't foolproof. You'll fall off from time to time if you're like most of us. But the act of creating it and referring to it to see how you are doing provides a discipline and language that helps you get back to the plan more quickly when you deviate from it.

I cannot over-emphasize the importance of having a plan for your health at the outset. Leadership work is a like a tsunami; if you don't prepare for its effects, you can be devastated when you experience them. It is hard to restore normalcy. You've already created expectations at the workplace, and you have a lot of ground to make up at home and with yourself. Build your plan ahead of time. At least have an idea of what you want to accomplish and how you will do it. Use it to create an understanding, even a contract, with your spouse and your family. Come back to it when you lose perspective and balance. Modify it as you gain experience. Like everything else, your health is a work in progress. Perceived this way, you and your family will want to find new ways that you can maintain your safe harbor, the alone time you need, the opportunities to take a deep breath and recharge your batteries, and at the same time maintain your focus on those most precious relationships you must have to succeed as a person and a leader.

PART TWO

PARTNERS

It takes a team to change your course. You need partners who are with you for the duration. If they are not, you will not succeed. It is as simple as that. Resistance, passive or active, will stall the changes, and the lack of on-the-ground knowledge and involvement will doom the effort to find and deliver the best care possible. Discovering and delivering superior care is not a job for outside experts or consultants; it requires the hands-on expertise of those who deliver the care either directly or in support roles, those who seek the care, and those along with you who are responsible for the health of the organization.

Several constituencies must be engaged for this to happen. First (chapter seven) are the patients, their families, those who depend on the services you provide, and the communities you serve. Your board of directors is a crucial ally too (chapter eight). Your leadership team and a broader leadership group help you shape, guide, and implement the changes (chapter nine). Obviously the partnership with the physicians is central to achieving any shifts in care delivery (chapter ten). But without the engagement of the entire workforce (chapter eleven), the changes will be incomplete, as the workforce—together with the physicians—provides the insights, innovations, and improvements that drive the quality of care higher. As important as the relationships are with each partner, they have even greater impact when they are formally codified into a written compact (chapter twelve).

CHAPTER SEVEN

THE HEART
OF THE MATTER

When the department chiefs and I met with representatives of several unions to discuss recent changes in our outpatient and inpatient care, the head of the local Longshoremen's Union asked when we planned to start evening and Saturday morning drop-in clinics to serve their members with families. The chiefs explained that they couldn't because the physicians were already fully scheduled and didn't have time. The questioner exploded, "We pay you! We're your customers. We've been asking you to do this for months. Our people need it. You gotta fix it." Others joined in. Tempers flared. It was tense and unpleasant. Finally the chiefs agreed to look into it, and within a few weeks, walk-in clinics were opened several evenings during the week and on Saturday mornings.

A similar experience occurred when a group of physicians and epidemiologists shared our proposed screening protocol for an hereditary form of breast cancer with an outside advocacy group. The advocates criticized the guidelines, accused us of withholding care to save money, and pointed out that our materials confused the patients, probably deliberately, with poorly written brochures and explanations. At first *our professionals were defensive and angry. But as other advocacy groups around the country expressed similar concerns, the physicians realized they needed to change their approach. They didn't alter the screening criteria, but rewrote the explanations and educational materials in collaboration with the advocacy groups. In turn the advocacy groups became public supporters of our approach. Because we sought their views, listened to what they said, and made a serious effort to incorporate their suggestions into the final product, we were able to establish a new level of trust and respect.*

Patients, family members, consumers of your services, and representatives of the communities you serve, can inspire, energize, goad, and even shame your organization as no others can. They are conversation-changers, focusing people on problems that matter, cutting through resistance, and rebalancing the power among those involved in delivering care. They are your heart, your most powerful partners in changing your organization, and used well, they can make magic happen.

Most of us track patient satisfaction through surveys and focus groups. But you need more than data to change your organization. You need the voices themselves. Impersonal survey data and second hand stories can be ignored, unpleasant findings rationalized, and the views of professionals can dominate. But face-to-face with the patients, when their voices surround you and they look you directly in the eye, the truth is hard to escape. This is what you want: their unfiltered, uncensored, unending stories reaching every nook and cranny of your organization, marinating it in the realities of those you serve.

Patients help you identify opportunities to improve their care, and when they do, the impact on your organization is profound. This should come as no surprise. They want the same things you do. They want their providers to care about them and offer safety and wise counsel, and they want high quality solutions that don't waste their time or their money. But the experience of receiving care is different from providing it. Like the play *Rashomon* in which individuals describe the same crime different ways, each constituent in your organization tells a different story about what goes on with care. Patients, physicians, other professionals, support people, and managers—everyone—bring a different insight and a unique sense of urgency to the care process. Your objective as the leader is to join these points of view, and especially important, to ensure that those of the patient are the main actors in the conversation.

How do you do it? How do you gain the full value of these voices and perspectives, create a patient- and consumer-centric culture in practice rather than in word? The impact you seek occurs because of a chorus of voices from many directions, addressing many problems over an extended period of time. It requires your steady and insistent leadership because it can be hard to get right. It can also be uncomfortable, especially at first, and often provokes resistance and outspoken criticism until it is firmly embedded in the way your organization operates every day.

So as you consider how to incorporate patients this way, be patient. Don't be too harsh on yourself or your organization. And don't give up. Your early attempts may be clumsy and not particularly successful. This is a new way to work for most of us; everyone has to learn as they go. The impact will grow as you gain experience. You can expect push back, especially from providers, because most aren't used to having direct conversations about what they do day in and day out, and few appreciate being confronted about shortcomings. This is exactly why these voices are so important. Those who serve and lead need to hear these stories, but it takes time to reach the point that they can. You have to help them get there.

During this learning process, you have to protect the patients from the experts, especially the physicians. You don't want them to be intimidated; they must be able to speak freely. They will need help to do this, to tell their stories effectively, understand what the ground rules are, and know what the expectations are for them and for others. And you need to guide those inside the organization as they learn to work with patients this way too: setting the ground rules, clarifying the underlying values, helping them honor these agreements, supporting them as they work at getting better at shared problem solving, and even disciplining those who refuse or are unable to do so.

At the same time, you have to insulate the organization from flamethrowers—those too consumed with anger or their own pain to be helpful. Patients will be selected for their stories, their personalities, and their ability to get noticed. At first, they will be the ones you know already, probably the most vocal. These aren't the wrong ones necessarily, but they can set back the effort if they aren't coached carefully. You must be careful not to derail the change effort by subjecting your organization and other patients to needless diatribes and personal vendettas.

You have to nurture this work too; the process and the participants must be managed carefully and funded appropriately. Consider assigning a senior manager to oversee the effort with the responsibility of identifying, preparing, and coaching the participants. That person also needs to keep an inventory of who has participated to ensure the reach is sufficiently broad and diverse. She should also have the responsibility of helping the entire organization learn how to work in partnership this way.

A patient- and consumer-centric partnership like this grows through actions at four levels within the organization: the individual patient experience; care delivery organization, design, and performance; organizational strategy; and community-centered health improvement efforts.

Level One: Patient-Care Experience

Multiple interventions are necessary to ensure that the patients' experiences with care are central to the care process itself. Think about:

AN ACTIVE PATIENT BILL OF RIGHTS

Walk into any clinic, emergency room, or hospital, and chances are you'll see a patient "Bill of Rights" posted somewhere. Some call it "Our Promise" or "Our Commitment" to you as the patient. These covenants usually say at least two things: every patient has the right to have the information she needs to make an informed decision about the care she receives, and every patient can expect to be treated with dignity and compassion. If this really happened, it would be exactly what we are looking for. The problem is that most organizations don't actively ensure that patients know what their rights are and how to exercise them. There are ways to change this. In addition to the routinely conducted patient satis-faction surveys, for example, you might consider the following:

- At the end of every care visit or episode, provide a written summary (at sixth grade reading level) of all decisions, immediate plans for further diagnostic work, agreed to therapies, and planned follow up. Assign a professional to review the materials with the patient and answer questions. Then as the first activity in the next outpatient visit or hospital rounds, determine what the patient and family are concerned about, and identify what was and was not done as planned. Repeat the process at every visit to an outpatient setting, and each day as part of regular rounds in the hospital. Record all changes in plans and failures to do what was planned into a database that can be used to help identify needed modifications in order sets, standard operating procedures, guidelines, and patient instructions.

- Conduct random in-person interviews with patients as they leave their clinic visit or await discharge from the hospital to determine whether or not they received instructions and understand them, and to assess how they were treated throughout their care. The results can be used to provide immediate feedback to clinicians, and to remediate poor communications and understanding. The information can be used to assess performance for purposes of improvement work, as well as to educate providers and support staff. The closer the feedback occurs to the actual patient experi-ence, and the more personal the feedback, the better.

- Train all professionals and support staff, especially physicians, in what the expectations are for how patients participate in their care and how they will be treated. Create performance standards based on these expectations, and use appropriate analytic tools to ensure that the standards are met. Even without a financial incentive, the act of clarifying, measuring, and giving feedback about information on performance reinforces the values you want to instill throughout the organization.

UBIQUITOUS STORIES

You want your patients and communities to be too powerful to ignore. Their stories should be part of all the conversations and dialogues that take place throughout the organization. You should fill your conversations with those stories too. The best, of course, are told by the patients. They may not speak well and the language may not be appropriate or easily understood, but it doesn't matter. These are *their* stories—good and bad, happy and sad. When they share their experiences with us, we can't help but think differently about what it means to be sick, what it is like to get care from us, and what we can do to make the lives of our patients better and healthier when they ask us for help. Here are some ways to begin.

- Start every board meeting with a patient story, preferably told by the patient. Limit the time to ten or fifteen minutes and leave time for questions. Help the patient prepare. Mix the stories—sometimes good, sometimes bad. After the patient leaves, discuss what you heard, learned, and how you plan to respond. Do the same thing at every senior team meeting, as well as other formal gatherings throughout the organization: all-hands meetings, orientation programs, and department meetings.

- Write a regular newsletter or e-mail for all employees and physicians that describes a patient experience and the organization's response.

- Create an organization-wide recognition program to honor teams that have worked effectively as partners with their patients to improve care.

DATA

Surveys and focus groups provide objective data on performance, complementing the anecdotal information you get from patients themselves. You need both to understand how well the organization and people within it meet your patient-centric care expectations. The simpler the better. Too much precision and detail are the enemy of effective feedback and learning. Frequency is important. If the data shows up once or twice a year, the surveys aren't worth the time and money. If data is a weekly stream, it overwhelms. There is no correct answer. You have to feel your way, combining the survey data with the anecdotes to build a culture of learning and improvement.

Level Two: Care Design, Improvement, and Accountability

Every care delivery design, improvement, and performance evaluation effort should include patients. For example:

TEAMS

Ensure that every team assigned to design, improve, or evaluate a care process or service includes at least two or more patients. For this to work as planned, you need to:

- Educate the patients about the problem they have been asked to address and how to participate on a team. Train the team members in working with patients. Help all team members, including patients, learn the tools and techniques for care design and improvement, and performance evaluation, consistent with the approaches you have chosen for your organization.

- Provide ongoing support with team management, provide feedback and coaching, and track progress on the assigned project.

SURVEYS AND FOCUS GROUPS

Every project should include survey data and, where possible, focus group data from patients to supplement the work carried out by the team. This way the insights of the patients on the team are combined with analytic data for a broad and robust assessment of patient preferences and needs.

Level Three: Strategic Planning

All strategic planning efforts should include patients, and, where possible, consumers and representatives from the community. Especially important are purchasers, e.g., employers, union trusts, and payers, for example. The goal is to build strategies that integrate the priorities of the patients and the community-based consumers of the services provided by the organization with those of the people of the organization. Consider the following:

- Organize your strategic planning efforts around teams that address specific problems, opportunities, and issues. Assign at least two to three patient and community representatives to each team.

- Roll up these efforts into the formal, overarching strategic plan to be reviewed by the senior management, the board of directors, and patient advisory councils (if present). If you don't have a patient advisory council, seek patient and community leader feedback in formal surveys and discussions, and in one on one conversations.

- Ensure that your final strategic goals for the organization are few. Three or four in a planning period is the maximum; two to three is more manageable.

Level Four: Community Health and Well-being

As you and your institution commit to enhancing the health and well-being of those who live in the communities you serve, you will want to join with others in this effort. Blending these voices creates the richest and most effective impact. You may wish to consider the following:

- Base these discussions on in-depth studies of the neighborhoods and sub-communities that make up the larger community in order to join stories and impressions with objective data for the ongoing programs you initiate.

- Support these community efforts with experts from your institution in clinical areas, and in team management and group problem solving. The community efforts are an opportunity to share the models and methods you've adopted in your own organization, and can help the deliberations move forward successfully.

- Engage your physicians and other clinicians in these discussions. This is valuable in two ways. First, they bring expertise to the discussions. Second, they learn from these experiences, and bring stories and insights about the needs and interests of the patients and community leaders back to their colleagues.

- Invite community leaders and patients to speak with your management teams and your board of directors about the community-based efforts, and in particular, the role the institution can play going forward.

You can readily see that a partnership with patients requires much more than patient advisory councils. They can be helpful, especially when they focus on a service or functional area within the organization, but councils alone aren't enough. Their voices are often muted, their passions and energies dulled by exposure to the ins and outs of the organization itself. You need more: a steady flow of creative, passionate, and fresh voices that reflect the immediate experiences of those you serve, and give urgency to the need to find ever-better solutions.

How will you know that you are building a patient- and consumer-centric culture? There is no good metric. You have to judge for yourself. You know you are on the right track if discussions of problems and challenges now include patients; if you and your senior team, managers, and clinicians routinely seek their voices to discover what works best; if patients report that they are included in conversations with their physicians about the clinical choices they have, and are given the final say in which decisions they make. If you see patients on every improvement team and design effort, and they are deeply involved in your strategic planning efforts, you are moving in the right direction. To be patient-

and consumer-centric as an organization requires that you maintain the active partnership at all levels as long as you are in the job. Without these voices, these perspectives, you risk "springing back" to the provider-centric culture of today.

CHAPTER EIGHT

BOARD OF DIRECTORS

It took several years before the KFHP/H board could carry out their fiduciary responsibilities effectively and function as a thought partner with the senior team and me. The shadows of the past haunted members who had served before I was named CEO. In spite of unanimous agreement that the organization needed to prepare for the challenges of the twenty-first century, it was hard for some of them to accept studies that were critical of organizational performance. And they were uncomfortable with any changes that threatened the stability of the Program. By 1994 the board membership had changed; several former officers of KFHP/H and individuals closely associated with the organization for many years had left. Those who remained were committed to building the new organization we needed. More than half were new; all former CEOs, leaders of their organizations, or experienced public company board members.

To educate them about the issues we faced, we increased the number of meetings from three to six, and devoted significant time at each meeting to reviewing the performance data and study results from the regional studies. We explored different ways to respond. Steadily the board grew to understand what the Program faced and what our choices were, and they played an increasingly active role in shaping our strategies and decisions. Because they were so deeply involved, they were steadfast in their support of me in spite of the ups and downs that occurred along the way.

The board of directors is your employer and alter ego. They hire, pay, and evaluate you; they terminate you if something goes wrong; and they name your successor when you leave. They stand side by side with you in leading the organization through the changes you will make. For your purposes, the best board will be one in which the members act as fiduciaries, moral stewards, thought partners, and ambassadors.

The fiduciary role is traditional for most boards, whether public, private, or not-for-profit. They are responsible for the integrity of financial reporting and for compliance with accepted accounting standards, as well as standards of behavior and honesty, and patient care. A board must act in good faith in its strategic decisions, its deployment of capital, and its decisions about the leadership of the organization. It must ensure that the organization carries out its legally mandated mission, a particularly important responsibility for 501(c)(3) organizations. The typical board is self-perpetuating and self-governing, choosing who sits on the board, who remains on the board, and how it conducts its business.

As moral steward, the board is especially important in helping you change your course. By law, the members are accountable for all care the patients receive, and for ensuring that the organization carries out its mission. This imposes a legal and ethical obligation that is distinct from that of the physicians or other clinicians. A physician is expected to act in the best interests of her patient and is legally accountable for the decisions and treatments she provides. The board, on the other hand, must protect all patients in the system and ensure that all decisions and treatments provided by all clinicians in the system are appropriate. The physician views her role in personal terms: she brings everything in her arsenal to help the patient in front of her; maintains her knowledge and her skills; secures more training and new skills as required; determines the limits of her competence throughout her career; establishes her referral network; and follows her own patients throughout the course of the conditions for which she is treating them. The board is responsible for the quality of every physician in the institution; oversees the design and function of the systems that enable patients to be served and safe; and monitors care and care processes to identify weaknesses and improvement opportunities.

These "clinical" and system imperatives must be balanced. Decisions made by the physician on behalf of a patient can harm the patient, the system, or both; decisions made to protect the system may ignore the needs of the individual patient. The board is the keeper of the system imperative. That is certainly its duty. At the same time, it must protect the patients and support the clinicians who make these difficult individual decisions every day. It is challenging to strike the right balance. The issues must be engaged again and again because there are no hard and fast rules. The tensions are never ending precisely because it is so difficult to find a permanent solution. The board functions at its highest moral level when it wrestles with these imperatives. Both are necessary to achieve the best possible care for each and all patients, the best solutions for each professional in the system, and all people who rely on the institution.

The board members also serve as your thought partners. This is a gift when you have the right people on your board. Whether you consult with them individually or as a full board, you benefit from their wisdom, experience, and perspectives. Like the gift that keeps on giving, the more familiar the board is with your plans, the more helpful they can be. A strong moral position about patient care, combined with helping you frame the changes the organization wishes to undertake, gives the board a powerful voice within the organization. You will need them as you confront the challenges and obstacles that lie on the path you have taken.

That said, it is not simple to establish this role of thought partner. You may be the most difficult hurdle of all. *You* may not want the board to interfere with your work. Perhaps you are content having them perform their fiduciary role, but otherwise, you want them as far away as possible from the messy, contentious decisions that you face. The board can be a hurdle too. They may not have sufficient trust in you or among themselves to engage in productive give and take discussions. One or two members may dominate, warping the dialogue and inhibiting participation. They may feel insecure dealing with clinical issues and physicians. These can be remedied if you plan carefully and are patient, and it is certainly worth the effort to do so.

To succeed as a community-based institution, you need to establish excellent relationships with constituents and resources outside the organization. The board can help you here too. Absorbed in daily responsibilities, it may be difficult for you to do this, to determine where and how to connect to the community, or how to establish the partnerships you need. The board can introduce you to people in their networks, and they can represent the institution in carrying out the community-directed work itself. They can also help you identify resources to support the changes you have begun in the organization. At Norton Healthcare, for example, CEO Stephen Williams and his board have invited non-healthcare experts in quality and quality improvement to contribute to the board's Quality Committee. This has the added advantage of introducing potential board members to the people of Norton Healthcare, and for board members to learn more about these candidates.

As you consider what kind of board you wish to develop, I would offer several recommendations.

Size and Structure

Smaller boards of nine to eleven members work better than larger ones. Fewer than nine and the workload can be overwhelming for the individual board members as they try to carry out their committee responsibilities and prepare for the regular board meetings. More than eleven members becomes challenging to make sure every person is well informed. There is also an upper limit for effective group discussion and problem solving. Once your board reaches twelve or more members, it starts to function as a collection of individuals rather than a cohesive unit. Unless required by law or regulation, no seat on a health system or hospital board should be "representative" of a particular group. The board's responsibility is to represent the community, the patients and consumers of the institution, and the institution itself; members should be the most highly qualified people available to do so, not the candidate of a particular constituency.

If you are able to build your own board, do not automatically include physicians. You may want their insights, but there are two dangers with including them on your board. First, your lay members may defer to them, making it harder to reach the appropriate balance you need between the clinical and system perspectives. Second, and more problematic, it can be harder to balance the interests of physicians with those of other important groups and constituents that make up your organization. But if your board has already developed the ability to support one another and function as a strong thought partner with you, the addition of a qualified physician, or even two, can further enrich its discussions and enhance the board's ability to carry out its work. If you do decide to include physicians, make sure each one you add meets the same standards as the other board members in terms of independence, integrity, experience, maturity, and the ability to work collaboratively with other board members.

You certainly want to include leaders with different backgrounds on your board. For example, individuals who are or have been CEOs of companies similar in size and complexity to your institution can provide helpful support. You should not limit your search just to people from the local communities you serve. With so much riding on regional and national developments, it can be helpful to include one or two experts from outside the community. You will also benefit by naming at least one person with a strong financial background, especially financial strategy (capital structure and deployment, balance sheet management, treasury functions), and control functions (accounting, audit, P&L integrity). Leaders with experience in quality management, particularly Lean or other highly developed quality disciplines, can transform the discussions. Experience in consumer goods marketing and sales outside of healthcare may also be useful. Someone with a background in human resources management will be a valuable advisor to you and a helpful contributor to the board. A person with experience in the political and regulatory institutions at the state or federal level can bring valuable insights about the increasingly government-centric world of healthcare.

It is often difficult to identify board candidates who mirror the ethnic backgrounds of the patients and communities you serve. The problem, in my experience, is not the availability of qualified candidates, but the difficulty reaching beyond familiar networks into other communities. As described later in the book, interest groups within the institution can help you with this. Whatever the hurdles, it is important to create a diverse board. The people who work in the institution should reflect the varied communities you serve. Patients and families want to see familiar faces when they seek your help. When your board reflects these same backgrounds, the bonds between your institution and the communities you serve are strengthened further. Diversity like this also adds bridges that help you work more closely with other leaders and patients from the neighborhoods and groups you serve. Most important, these different points of view enrich the deliberations of the board as you work through the tough decisions you face.

Finally, a word about whether or not your predecessor should remain on the board after stepping down as CEO. In general this is a poor governance practice no matter how helpful or knowledgeable the individual might be. An argument can be made to have the former CEO continue in the role of chairman of the board for a transition period of a few months where there is no suitable independent chairman candidate to serve in that role or when the new CEO will eventually become the chairman of the board. The central argument for not including the predecessor on the board after she steps aside is that she tends to inhibit the incumbent in making needed changes, adding new perspectives, or even gathering information to help identify where problems and opportunities lie within the organization. The predecessor's shadow is large and makes it difficult for a board and an incumbent to find the daylight they need to move ahead. The transition period of a few months may be useful to give the incumbent an opportunity to become established as CEO without the added burden of dealing with board governance. If this model is used, it is important to ensure that the timeline is clear, and that the predecessor's role is proscribed: she needs to focus just on governance and managing the meetings. The CEO should be able to set the agenda and prepare the materials. The interim chairman's position is designed to facilitate the transition of the CEO into the chairman's role, not continue to control the agenda or direction of the organization.

Contracts and Compacts

Not-for-profit hospitals and health systems have, for the most part, asked volunteers to serve on their boards. The responsibilities of the board may be outlined in the bylaws, but the conventions for how the board operates are often shared informally, from a sitting board member to an incoming one. There may be an orientation session or two, but performance expectations are often not high, and significant education and preparation is not considered appropriate or necessary.

This is a mistake. Your healthcare institution is probably a multi-million dollar business with a complex mission. You need a hardworking, committed, and effective board to help you lead it. While an unpaid, volunteer board can sometimes do this—as many high-performing examples demonstrate—you increase the likelihood that your board will function at the level you require if you establish a paid relationship with them, an effective orientation system, and a formal evaluation process.

- If you have a foundation or a similar vehicle for making financial contributions to the community, you can provide each board member with a specified match to his or her charitable contributions to qualified 501(c)(3) organizations that meet specifications you delineate. At Kaiser Permanente, for example, we originally matched such contributions on a three to one basis (we contributed three dollars for every dollar a board member contributed) up to a limit of $30,000 per year. The current policy is to provide a one to one match. Eligibility continues after stepping down from the board based on the years of service; one year of continued eligibility for every year served, up to ten years. A similar policy existed when I served on the Rockefeller Foundation Board of

Trustees. Many for-profit companies provide matching grants at different levels as well.

- You may wish to pay a token retainer in return for board service. You can supplement this with meeting fees, though this complicates the administration of the program. There is no ideal amount for the retainer. It depends on what you are allowed to pay, and what you can afford. A helpful rule of thumb, I found, was to keep the annual total at no more than 10 percent of the average annual retainer and fee total for comparably sized private and public companies in your area. If you keep compensation at this relatively modest level, you are unlikely to encounter resistance from the community, or run into political criticism. The value of the retainer rests with the implicit contract it establishes between the institution and each individual on the board. This agreement, combined with an explicit compact (see below) that details expectations, provides a stronger foundation for a constructive working relationship than a purely volunteer model can.

- You and your board can establish an explicit agreement, what the board of Virginia Mason Health System calls a "compact," that details the expectations the board has for its members and the institution, and in return, what the institution and you can expect from the board. This formalization can be helpful when recruiting new members for the board, and it helps for evaluating and improving board performance and relationships between the board and the institution and you as the leader.

- You should evaluate the board on a regular basis. This should include an assessment of the board as a whole; ideally it includes an evaluation of each member as well. It doesn't matter whether or not the members are paid or in some way rewarded for their service, they deserve feedback about their performance as seen through the eyes of their colleagues. This can be done informally in confidential conversations between the board chair and each member, or in a formal, confidential, and written evaluation process that everyone participates in. You can ask for qualitative assessments that are open-ended, or you can design a numerical evaluation system if you prefer. You may want to conduct an evaluation of every member each year, or you can focus on those whose terms are up for renewal and in the course of three to four years complete evaluations of every board member. Whatever the model, it is valuable to "close the loop" with each individual in a private conversation. Like the evaluations of the people who report to you, these should be candid, and constructive. If there is a significant performance problem, this is the time to deal with it. When a board member is not pulling her weight, she needs to improve or be asked to step aside.

Leadership and Terms of Service

The CEO position in a healthcare institution is a demanding job, and getting more so all the time. That of board chairman faces escalating challenges too. If possible, the two roles should be separated. The CEO has more than enough work to lead the institution; the chairman of the board needs to focus on providing the highest possible level of support and oversight. Moreover, the more independent the board is perceived to be, the greater its influence in helping drive the organization forward.

The question of board terms remains unsettled. There is no particular value in rotating the chairmanship of the board. The goal, after all, is to have a high-performing board, not one that is "democratic" or "representational." It is valuable to establish terms of office for each board member—typically three years—with the opportunity to be reappointed for additional terms, usually three terms or a total of nine years of service. This provides the board and the chairman with the opportunity to evaluate each board member on a scheduled basis, provide feedback designed to improve individual effectiveness, and in rare cases, ask a person to leave the board. It also lets you refresh the board with new perspectives and skills as board members rotate off. The chairman of the board should be evaluated on the same schedule that you are evaluated as

CEO. If the board as a whole determines that a change in leadership is required, the chairman should be replaced.

Meetings

Your overriding priority is to change the direction of your institution. Every board meeting should focus on progress, obstacles, issues, and improvements related to this objective. Each, as noted, should begin with stories from patients. Key fiduciary and change milestones should be tracked at each meeting. Every meeting should have some educational component, typically focused on a department or improvement effort within the institution. Fiduciary matters should be the last item on the agenda, not the first; you want to be sure to focus most on the strategic and operational issues related to the transformation. The exception is when a significant fiduciary problem arises, in which case it must be given sufficient time for review and decisions. Reports should be distributed in writing in advance whenever possible, and discussions during the meetings should summarize key points, allow for questions, and lead to actions. Wherever possible, formal presentations should be avoided, replaced with more freewheeling discussions instead.

- A standard "decision format" for the board is helpful. For example, you may want to summarize a problem in writing, explain why it is important, describe the options, and present your recommendation in a standard presentation format. Some boards limit these decision-memos to three to five pages. Commonly the decision process begins with a review at the relevant board committee, moves forward on their recommendation, and then is reviewed with the full board for final action. Or you can do it in two or three steps with the full board: at the first meeting discuss the problem, the options, and the recommended action; at the second, review comments, reactions, and proposed action; at the third, take formal action. You can shorten this any way you wish. Establishing a predictable rhythm is important to make sure that the board and inside leaders are not taken by surprise and have sufficient opportunity to participate.

Some boards meet monthly, others each quarter. The first is too frequent; it is difficult to prepare properly in this kind of time frame, and doing so places a heavy and distracting burden on you and your senior leadership team. Boards then tend to become too deeply involved in daily operations. Quarterly meetings may not be frequent enough. For a board member to learn enough to be helpful requires continuity and relatively frequent immersion through discussions at the board meetings. A good compromise is to have six scheduled meetings a year, adding others as necessary.

A well-organized board meeting should not take more than half a day. It is helpful to schedule one longer meeting or retreat per year that combines strategic planning and a deeper examination of the most pressing issues the organization faces. A retreat like this can help build the capabilities of the board and the trust between senior management and the board through formal and informal interactions.

Committee Structure

The work of the board and the organization of the committees should reflect your transformation imperative. Your goal is to minimize the time board members spend on their fiduciary obligations while protecting the integrity of the institution. You want to be sure to devote considerable board time to two major committees that reflect key elements of the new capacities you are building: (1) the execution of the quality improvement effort within the institution, including regular review of quality improvement results; and (2) the development and execution of overall change strategy and performance, including key human resources, culture and organizational change efforts, market share changes, and longer term positioning. Every board member should serve on one of these two committees. It is also helpful to add outside experts to these committees. This serves two purposes. Outside experts broaden the perspectives and deepen expertise, and they develop a relationship with the institution that can lead to an appointment to the parent board when the opportunity arises. Often they will serve voluntarily, although, as with the board members, you may wish to provide them with some sort of de facto contract in the form of a charitable matching program, or something similar.

Most boards delegate finance, audit, governance, and compensation responsibilities to committees; the results are reported at each board meeting of the whole. You can choose to combine committees, for example audit and finance. You can carry out governance functions as a committee of the whole. Compensation issues, which primarily involve the evaluation of the CEO and setting her compensation, as well as establishing compensation policy and reviewing major compensation decisions for the institution, can be done once a year in a committee or as a board, with ad hoc decisions in the interim as necessary.

Your board is a crucial asset in your efforts to transform your organization. Their moral authority as fiduciaries for the institution and as representatives of patients and the communities you serve is an important counterbalance to the perspective that physicians have traditionally brought to healthcare institutions. Their insights can help you formulate the best solutions and most appropriate approaches to the transformation you lead, while their support can help you make the hard choices and implement the difficult changes that lie ahead.

CHAPTER NINE

THE SENIOR LEADERSHIP TEAM

AND

THE CHANGE LEADERSHIP NETWORK

I once recruited an experienced leader into the organization and over time assigned her increasingly broader responsibilities. Her performance deteriorated with each new assignment. It wasn't just her performance. Concerns also emerged about her management style, her treatment of subordinates, and her tendency to set one senior team member against another. Through it all, though, I remained stubbornly committed to her, and spent considerable time counseling her about her leadership and performance shortcomings. I was convinced she had what it takes, and that I could teach her to lead and motivate others to achieve the performance we needed. Only when several members of the senior team expressed their concerns to me in private conversations did I take off my blinders. My colleagues were right. She wasn't the right person for the job, and she'd begun to compromise the integrity and credibility of the team itself. I had to let her go, and I'd already waited longer than I should have to do so.

It is sobering to realize how long I rationalized like this. It happened several times with team members I inherited when I began, and also with people I had promoted or recruited. It isn't an uncommon problem. Jack Welch, the hard-nosed former leader of General Electric, once told me he "wouldn't have waited so long to change people I knew couldn't do the job." Although never a pushover when it came to hiring and firing people, he admitted that he deluded himself into believing he could change people through counseling, support, and expectation setting. Other leaders with whom I have spoken describe similar experiences.

Sometimes the issue isn't waiting too long. It is not knowing enough to realize what skills, perspectives, and, most importantly, complementarity between you and a particular team member are missing. In one instance, the shortcomings became obvious only after a team member left for personal reasons, and the person I recruited to fill the position turned out to be a better fit for the organization and for me.

Waiting too long is the more common problem, though. We try everything to fix the situation and, more often than not, end up asking the person to leave the organization anyway. It is painful to make the final call, and it should be. These are your teammates, after all, the people you've worked with over many long hours and days, even months and years.

It shouldn't be easy to ask someone to leave, especially when the reasons involve performance or fit instead of something egregious like fraud or inappropriate behavior. I agonized each time to be sure I was making the right call, and that the person was being treated with dignity and respect. It was important not just to be consistent with my own values, but also because the way people leave sends such a strong message throughout the organization about how people are valued.

I learned an important lesson about this early in my career when the head of the largest department in the organization I led at the time lied to my face, and I fired him on the spot. Although his job performance warranted the firing and he needed to go, I didn't handle the situation with the care it needed. I continued to see him in social settings as our children attended the same schools and our colleagues knew us both. He was also a highly visible and well-respected healthcare leader with deep ties to the political establishment in our jurisdiction that he immediately called upon to fight my decision. A hue and cry in the local press brought unwelcome visibility to the organization and the leadership team. We had a messy, unpleasant divorce because of my impulsive, emotional handling of the situation. It was an important lesson: the macho approach to leadership in which you fire someone on the spot without regard for the impact on the organization, the downstream consequences, and most of all, the rules of decency and civility, has no place in the world I wanted to be part of. It is also anathema to building the trust and confidence one needs to lead these complex organizations we serve.

Two distinct groups are required to help you lead the changes in your organization. First is the senior leadership team responsible for the performance of the organization as a whole. This group is named by the CEO, often approved by the board of directors, and represents the formal C-suite of officers and leaders for the organization. It has two accountabilities: to make sure the organization operates successfully day in and day out, and to help you implement the new capabilities.

A second group is a network—larger, amorphous, shifting, and changing over time—which includes individuals whose leadership can help move the course change forward. Potential members of this second group are thought leaders among clinicians and support staff, individuals from outside the organization who live in the community and are leaders in their own right, and people whose special skills are important at one point or another in the course of the transformation. Some, perhaps all, of the senior leadership team can join the larger group. From time to time, you may want to appoint an especially effective thought leader to the senior leadership team in a permanent role.

THE SENIOR LEADERSHIP TEAM

The senior leadership team is the small group you work with every day. It should include a mix of perspectives, styles, skills, and backgrounds that complement your own and help you find a well-rounded view of what needs to happen for the organization to succeed. Its members share the values and the same deep commitment to the patients and workforce that you do, but bring distinct voices and may offer different views about how to solve the problems and challenges. As you think about how to build your team, you want to consider several points.

Make Up

As noted earlier, Abraham Lincoln was a moral and empathetic leader whose intellect and independence helped him work with those around him. He knew his limits and wanted to be sure he considered other points of view. The individuals on his team had their own constituents; their webs of influence complemented his so the reach of the team exceeded that of any single individual on it.

This is a key consideration as you construct your team. Which individuals complement you? You do not want people with incompatible values about how to treat people or how to lead others, nor do you want individuals who fail to share your central purpose. But you do need people around you who challenge your thinking, who bring other perspectives about what needs to happen and how to do it. You want them to have their own networks throughout the organization and beyond that they can draw upon to extend the lines of communications about what the organization is doing and why. I can't overemphasize this. It is a mistake to surround yourself with people who think like you do, and who are easy for you to be with. You benefit most when real differences exist and decisions are strongly debated. This is how you make sure the decisions are sound. You do whatever analysis you can to develop an "objective" view of what the choices and consequences might be. Then you look for the real meat behind these analyses—the tensions and realities that don't emerge until you and your team feel them, stew on them, argue over them, and work through the best and worst possible outcomes. Good decisions combine careful analysis and vigorous debate. This doesn't mean you have to pull hair and rip clothes. We're not talking about the sarcastic, point-scoring political battles you see in the Knesset in Israel, or the House of Commons in the United Kingdom. You are with your team day in and day out, handling tough issues all the time. You need a safe place for productive discussions, where respect and civility are required, where different points of view are listened to and sought, where the gentlest on the team can argue with the loudest and most difficult, where every person on the team feels as though her views matter and she is respected and safe. Your job is to construct your team with these different perspectives, then lead in such a way that these views can surface in the team's discussions.

You have to know your own flat spots inside and out to ensure that your team provides what you cannot. Before you put your team together, you should take your own assessment of what you do well and what you don't, what you like and what you don't, and what you are likely to see clearly and where your blind spots lie. Most of us already know these things, at least to some extent. But now is the time for brutal honesty, no holds barred. Your success as a leader is dependent in significant measure on how well you put your team together. You may want someone to help you with this process, an advisor, a consultant, or a friend, as they see you from a different perspective. Once you have the information, you are in the best position to create the most well-rounded team possible.

There are three positions that every team must have: chief financial officer, human resources leader, and chief information officer. Other positions will reflect the stage of development of the organization, its unique requirements, and its history. You may want a chief operating officer, a chief medical officer, or a chief of nursing. You may include your chief counsel on the team. You get the idea. Your organizational structure and the membership of the team depend on you and your circumstances. Beyond the CFO, HR leader, and the CIO, it is an open field.

Why a CFO? The most obvious reason is to protect you and the organization from financial problems that arise either in the course of daily operations or from changing your course. You need someone to keep the books, do the projections, follow the trends, and assess the results, someone who is compulsive, good at making sure this happens, and whose attention to detail frees you to focus where you need to. She should have the intelligence, experience, and maturity to interpret the numbers and help you and the rest of the team understand what is happening financially and where you might be heading. She should be good at identifying what is important in order to avoid wasting time chasing down false alarms.

But this is only part of what a good CFO provides. Your CFO should be a leader too, someone who thinks strategically about the business and looks beyond the month or year to assess where things could go in the future. She needs to read the tea leaves. She also helps define your financial strategy: your capital structure, use of capital, and access to capital. She is the front person with the lending agencies if you borrow to finance your major acquisitions, new buildings or technologies. She puts realistic boundaries on what might happen if you choose one path or another. She is your guru for creating realistic "if-then" financial scenarios that you must have to lead responsibly. Finally, it helps if she can communicate these ideas so that non-financial people understand them.

CFOs like this do not come along every day. They do not have to come from inside healthcare, although it helps with all the ins and outs of the reimbursement systems, payers, provider contracts, and regulations you deal with. Many leaders undershoot with their CFO choices, selecting good accountants to perform the control functions, but not a financial strategic partner or leader. It's a dangerous deficit. You can shore up this weakness in the short term by asking a member of the board with strong financial credentials to mentor your CFO. You may even ask that person to play a more active role in leading the board's financial committee and review of operations and decisions. For the longer term, however, there is no substitute for a strong CFO who works side by side with you every day.

What about the HR leader? In many organizations, the HR leader is a policeman, the enforcer of myriad rules and regulations about how people are treated and paid. She makes sure the paychecks get out on time. This is too narrow. The HR leader is responsible for these basics. That's a given. But she also helps you engage and train your workforce, and prepare leaders in the organization to support your course-change agenda, including the partnerships with patients and communities. She helps you develop the board of directors, and your accountability and incentive programs to support your long-term goals. An outstanding HR leader will put these in place, at the same time providing you and your team a unique perspective on the progress of the transformation, how the workforce is doing, what the impact on morale is, how stressed they are, and what kind of leadership interventions are required. An added bonus is when the HR leader can be a trusted, behind-the-closed-door advisor to you and to the others on the leadership team. With the right combination of insight, maturity, and respect, she can be the go-to person for these private discussions, especially about interpersonal issues, team building, and career planning.

The CFO and HR leader play similar roles then. Both must build strong organizations to protect the integrity of the organization. Both are strategic; they provide analysis and understanding regarding what resources—financial and personnel—will be required to accomplish what you seek, and they know how to get things done. Both must communicate effectively throughout the organization so that logic and discipline of appropriate human and financial capital use are an integral part of the new culture. And both advise you. They must be able to share their ideas and insights with you, and you must trust and respect them highly enough to listen.

The third named player is the Chief Information Officer. Information is the lifeblood of the modern healthcare system, built on a combination of modern data capture and communications technologies, complex analytics, and old-fashioned face-to-face communications and problem solving. The goal of your course change is for patients, clinicians, and support staff to communicate with one another anytime, anywhere, and to share information that makes care more effective and safe. To do this requires real-time, transparent information about performance, readily available for any kind of leadership discussion. You have to know how you are doing compared to the goals you've set, whether or not you are getting better, whether or not patients are safer and better treated. The CIO builds and maintains the systems that make this happen. And, like the CFO and HR leader, she must help the organization understand where the field is moving and how to get there. She, too, is both strategic and operational. She works with the patients, clinicians, and support staff to determine what information is important, then helps you create the infrastructure for making this a reality. Beyond this, the CIO should help you and your leadership team understand where the field is moving, both in terms of information and communications, and in the rapidly evolving world of data analytics in patient care. We'll explore this further in chapter seventeen.

If, for whatever reason, you are unable to recruit individuals with the requisite strategic, forward-thinking capabilities in the CFO, HR leader, and CIO roles, you should not include them on your senior leadership team. Individuals who cannot elevate above their control and day-to-day management functions are a drag on senior leadership performance, often inhibiting the creative work of building the new culture. It is better to have them report to a senior leader who possesses the requisite flexibility to manage the operational and transformational levels.

What happens if someone doesn't work out as a member of your team? Most leaders wait too long to act when someone is unable to perform as expected. You will probably struggle with these issues, and agonize over these decisions. I hope you do because these are some of the toughest calls you must make. They involve someone you know well, after all, often a person you have relied on and care about. You have to encourage the individual to reach the level of performance and participation you need. But once you know she is not right for your team, you have to act. You cannot delay, because the team becomes tainted, its weakest link exposed to the rest of the organization.

Acting like this isn't difficult when someone is unethical, or when she does not embody the values you have agreed to. There are rarely extenuating circumstances that justify these lapses. Sometimes counseling is the right answer, especially when a person has no prior history, or when the failure is a relatively minor one. But rest assured that people in the organization either know already or will soon find out what has occurred. They watch to see if you are serious about the values you espouse. More often than not in such circumstances, the right answer is to ask the person to leave. As important as it is to act, the way you carry out the decision is just as important. She must be able to leave with as much dignity and sensitivity as possible under the circumstances. The rest of the organization needs to understand what has happened, and you should not be afraid to explain so they can. It's an important "teachable moment" for the organization too. At the same time, you have to convey the message that people matter, and they will be treated with dignity and compassion, even when they can no longer be part of the organization. It is a tough line to walk and an important test of your leadership.

I've described the makeup of the senior leadership team in terms of the diversity of perspective and skills required to create a well-rounded group that complements your strengths and weaknesses. Another aspect of diversity deserves special mention. You may serve a diverse population in terms of race, religion, culture, language, and origins. Current demographic trends suggest that we will be a nation of minorities by the year 2050; several states already are. This poses a real challenge for a healthcare system that seeks to be patient centered.

We know that different ethnic groups have distinct clinical needs and bring unique expectations and values to their encounters with health professionals and the system. We know too that clinical outcomes, or health status, vary among different groups. These disparities have been the focus of numerous studies over the past two decades. We also know that language has an important impact on the quality of the interactions with health professionals and institutions. If you have ever been sick in a country whose language and culture is not yours, you know how difficult it can be to get the care and the comfort you need.

How can we respond? Building an organization that reflects the people and cultures of the communities you serve is both a moral and competitive imperative. Focus on your senior leadership team and your board of directors. It is not easy to do so, however. You must be creative in your searches and recruiting to find a pool of qualified candidates for these leadership roles. It's also slow; you build a reputation for your commitment to diversity one step at a time.

Dynamics

Your responsibility is to help the team develop, particularly its problem-solving and creative capabilities. You have to encourage everyone to participate—highlighting the differences, testing alternative hypotheses, and shaping and articulating agreements when possible. You need to be clear about when a decision will be reached by consensus and when it is yours.

You may be tempted to avoid difficult, emotional discussions by playing the role of an independent arbiter among members of your team who disagree. You might be tempted to act as a broker or nego-tiator to find a compromise that can work for everyone. This is a debili-tating and eventually destructive approach to leadership. Most difficult discussions need to take place with everyone in the room. Creating side channels is time consuming and robs the team of the opportunity to share passions and points of view that build common purpose over time. Conflicts can get out of hand, of course. A strong personality can overwhelm someone who is more reluctant to engage. It isn't always possible to reach agreement. You may have no choice but to broker an agreement, especially for a highly contentious issue. It isn't wrong, but it can become harmful if it is your main approach for dealing with issues like these.

It is common wisdom that your leadership team should be "on the bus" with you, that there must be "no space" among you when you take a decision into the organization. Once a decision is made, it shouldn't be changed. You might believe that conflict among members of your leadership team encourages disagreements and divisions within the organization. Be careful. Some decisions are final—you buy a hospital, invest in a technology, create a new program, or fire a manager. Many other decisions, in fact I would suggest most of them, are the best you can do with the information you have at the time. Decisions like these unfold over time as new information and insights emerge that cause you to shift and change directions. You'd be ill advised not to. Staying the course can become nothing more than blind stubbornness. You actually want more information, more ideas, more perspectives, and the push and pull of different arguments. To reach the right decision in situations like this requires flexibility, like the open-field runner in a football game, the ability to dodge and weave on the way to the end zone. When you deal with a cut-and-dried decision, you want the leadership team to present a unified front. When decisions are the best you can do with the information you have, as most are, you want disagreement and discussion. You want the leadership team to communicate the decision and learn and adjust as the decision is rolled out. You want members of the leadership team with different points of view to encourage others in the organization to express their own. You want an engaged workforce actively discussing and debating, disagreeing even, sharing different ideas and solutions because there is no "right" answer. You want to convey that the goal is to learn, get better, rather than to make a decision and stubbornly refuse to acknowledge new information or ideas that can improve it.

It is important for your team to be loyal to the institution and to the leadership team. They need to be committed to what you are trying to accomplish, to the quest for superior care for patients. They need to be loyal to the idea that they owe it to one another to tell the truth and express their points of view in order to be a better leadership team. You cannot have people on your team who actively sabotage you or their teammates at every opportunity. Backstabbing and passive aggressive behavior has no place on a team or organization built on the principle of mutual respect. It's a cancer that has to be eliminated.

Organization

The organization of your senior leadership team changes with your needs as a leader and those of the organization itself. In the beginning, it is probably wise to have a flatter structure with more people reporting directly to you. This helps you learn about the organization and be more directly involved in the management and changes underway.

With time you may wish to focus on the capacity building efforts for the organization and leave the daily operations to others. It makes sense then to have a smaller group of direct reports, even as few as two or three, each with a larger span of responsibilities reporting to them. There's always a trade-off. By inserting two or three people between you and the rest of the organization, you risk losing touch with day-to-day operations. You can overcome this by devoting your time to working in the organization on the daily improvement efforts. You can also use the senior team meetings to make sure you and everyone else is grounded in what is going on in daily operations.

In the final analysis, there is no "right" structure. It is important to stay flexible, to be willing to experiment and shift direction as you learn, grow, and change. But remember, an organization can take only a finite amount of change. Changes at the top are particularly unsettling; they require people to rethink relationships and roles, and learn new ways to get things done. Exercise flexibility with caution. Too little change and the team may fail to grow with the organization itself. Too much and the organization can become unstable for a period of time while attention shifts from the real work to trying to figure out how to get things done in a new structure.

Meetings and Retreats

How often to meet and how to organize the meetings is a matter of personal preference. Regularly scheduled meetings are important, a checking-in and information sharing that keeps you in the loop and the leadership team functioning smoothly. While these should be focused, short and to the point, this discipline cannot get in the way of real-time discussions or decisions when an issue requires it. When you act as issues arise, you create a sense of urgency in your team and the rest of the organization. People don't have to wait for answers, and they see that action matters. Meetings that take place on-site together with the people doing the daily work also drive your changes forward. Not only do you and your team see things firsthand, those on the front lines learn that you support them on concerns that matter to them. If you can, try to resolve any problems that come up in these meetings immediately, on the spot, especially if they are organizational barriers and policies that inhibit daily work and ongoing improvement efforts. To make changes happen, you want to create a sense of urgency, focus, and collaboration within the organization. On-site meetings are an excellent opportunity for you to model the behavior you want, especially the shared problem-solving, engagement, discussion, and debate that energizes the workforce and makes full use of their talents.

Use other gatherings for more complex, problem-solving, and strategic explorations that require analysis and consideration of distinct options, as well different points of view. These are particularly useful when you and your team need to challenge assumptions or rethink the way you are doing things. For these to work effectively, you must create an atmosphere conducive to reflection, a safe harbor for the discussion, disagreements, and conflicts that often surface in these circumstances. A day or two away from the office is helpful, especially if you can find somewhere relaxed to meet. Much can get done in settings like this, especially if they are meticulously planned.

That raises a final point. You need to be sure that the background materials, the analyses, and the presentations are up to standard and support long-term objectives for every agenda item. Data needs to be accurate and well organized, options fleshed out, and recommendations clearly articulated. Questions for discussion require planning too. Pre-meeting get-togethers are often useful, especially one-on-one sessions to explore the issues, find out what is on the mind of the individual, and begin to identify the potential conflicts and areas of agreement. As mentioned earlier, you don't want to fall in the trap of trying to resolve these issues during these one-on-one discussions. Rather you want to know enough in advance to be able to structure the discussions to have the greatest likelihood of a productive outcome. Similar to board discussions, a standard presentation format that applies to a range of problems can be helpful. It should be focused and concise, contain only the data required to understand the problem, the options to consider, the pros and cons of each, and the recommended choice and why. This discipline and rhythm to decision-making and option-consideration improves quality and keeps you and the team from drowning in the cacophony of daily problems and challenges in a typical healthcare system.

THE CHANGE LEADERSHIP NETWORK

This is a patchwork quilt of thought leaders, critics, confidants, influencers, strong thinkers, and experts selected to help you and your senior leadership team move your course-change agenda forward. Some may be important spokesmen for the current culture; others may push for change. Some may be thoughtful loners whose insights about performance open minds; others may be effective at motivating those around them. You need a combination to shape your agenda and move the improvement processes deep into the organization. You need people who are willing to give you unwelcome news, and tell the truth about how things are going, both good and bad. You want the rest of the organization to see the people they respect and trust join you to push ahead with the new capabilities you are building.

This network is a living organism. It is likely to change shape and composition, expand and contract, and shift focus over time as the agenda moves ahead. While there may be a core of change leaders throughout the process, your network should evolve in response to the challenges you face during your journey. It may never be a formal group, though in the interests of transparency, the sooner the organization knows who is involved the better. To start the process, you want to identify individuals you might want to involve, then meet one on one to learn what concerns they have, how they think and communicate, and how they might work with others. Some will be helpful in one-on-one discussions but difficult in groups. Others may be reluctant to talk in groups but provide valuable insights in private conversations. Still others support the transformation and should be visible in the effort because of their formal or informal leadership roles in the organization. You bring people into the network as you find and need them, you meet with them in whatever way maximizes their impact, and you recognize them in ways that respond to their needs and yours. The individuals may not need formal titles or assignments. They may become members of your senior leadership team but don't have to. It can be helpful to provide the more active among them with a compensation adjustment to recognize the time they invest beyond (or instead of) their regular income generating activities. All of this is flexible. There is no right way, only the recognition that a network like this is an essential building block for effective design and implementation of what you want to accomplish.

Among the most important members of your leadership network are the formal and informal physician thought leaders and critics. In the next chapter we'll discuss how to identify and engage these leaders, and more broadly, how to encourage the physicians to become the advocates for changes that, on the surface, appear to run counter to their established culture and economic interests.

CHAPTER TEN

PHYSICIANS

The young gastroenterologist sitting next to me fell asleep at least three times during the speeches and shoptalk at dinner. The leaders of the community hospital were animated, and so were most of the other local physicians around the table. But he was exhausted. During a lull in the conversation, I asked if he'd had a tough night on call the night before. He shook his head. It wasn't about a patient, he explained. He and his partner were in the process of merging with another three-person GI group. The five of them had met from seven p.m. until well after midnight the night before to work through the logistics of their new group. The last two hours were spent arguing over the letterhead on their new stationery. They couldn't agree and left. "This group practice stuff is really hard." He said wearily. "We can't agree on anything. I don't know if we can pull it off."

It is challenging to lead physicians. We seldom agree on anything, resist rules and discipline, and fight change. I once believed that with enough patience, sound reasoning, and good process, it was always possible to reach a consensus. I've long since changed my view. A leader has to know when there is enough consensus to make a decision without having things blow up, be sure to prepare for things to blow up anyway, and understand that some subset of the physicians will always be angry no matter how good your groundwork. You have to keep moving forward, undeterred by the emotional, often personal attacks that are so common among us.

You have no choice. You cannot deliver the best care possible without your physicians. The changes cannot be imposed, nor can non-clinicians or outsiders make them happen. Financial incentives will not do it either. Physicians have to be persuaded to leave behind the culture they have been immersed in since they decided to enter the profession. They have to agree to help design the new one, and then they must continuously improve what they've put in place. For you to convince them to do these things, you have to understand why it is so difficult for them to do so.

Resistance to change is a predictable outgrowth of how physicians are trained, and the status they enjoy. They are shaped by a powerful socialization system, strong ethical constraints, laws and regulations, economic incentives, and the expectations of their patients and the public. They are at the top of the medical hierarchy by tradition and law, and compensated accordingly. It is no surprise that they are slow to embrace change; they have the most to lose.

Selection into medical school is highly competitive. Prospective students must meet difficult academic requirements and perform well on the Medical College Admission Test (MCAT). In spite of these hurdles, the individuals admitted to medical school are, in the main, an idealistic lot. An intense education and socialization process begins on day one of medical school. Mastery is the goal: the science that underlies medical decision-making and the myriad skills of clinical practice. The student is also immersed in medical ethics. She learns about them from her professors, sees them in practice, witnesses their breech when patients are mistreated, and is constantly reminded of them as she hones her own capabilities.

The focus on mastery and ethics provides a powerful socialization into the profession. The student learns how to care for many different patients by watching and doing, seeing senior physicians solve clinical problems, and then doing it herself. She learns how to act and how to be a physician by working next to the senior physicians, the faculty, and resident staff who teach and oversee her work. Day after day, month after month, and year after year, this is drummed into her. To graduate, to take the Hippocratic Oath, she must have mastered the judgments, the skills, the ethics, and the behaviors that define her profession.

Residency training requires from three to seven or eight years more study after medical school to become qualified for specialty practice. Today most physicians who want to practice pursue some specialty preparation; the experience is narrower, deeper, and the socialization is even more intense than in medical school. Again the physician learns by doing, by taking care of patients. She works under the direction of senior physicians, gaining greater independence each year, until in the last phase, she supervises younger physicians-in-training and provides care with minimal supervision. She may follow residency with a one to two year fellowship that focuses on research and even more highly sub-specialized patient care, usually in the protective cocoon of an academic medical center or research institution.

After those two to four years of pre-medical studies, four years of medical school, three to seven years of residency training, and perhaps a fellowship of one to two years, she emerges as a highly trained, specialized physician with deeply ingrained habits and beliefs. She has learned to rely on herself, her own judgments, to function autonomously, to trust her work and be skeptical of the work of others. She has learned what her obligations are to her patients and her colleagues, and how to meet them. She has learned many tricks—habits—that help her manage her time and marshal the mental and physical energy to deal with the intense and unending demands of caring for difficult patients with challenging problems. She has also learned to be in charge and function at the top of the hierarchy. At each rung in her development, her influence, power, and status has grown. But she has learned little about the economics of medical care, including how she will make a living as a physician.

She may have talked with physicians in practice. She may even have a glancing familiarity with the way her professors are paid through their practice plan. If she is like most, though, she has little exposure to medical economics, different payment systems, or ways to organize her practice. In fact, during a decade or more of preparation, she has devoted virtually all of her energies to learning how to care for her patients the way she is expected to, and building the decision-patterns, the skills, the judgments, and the habits that enable her to do so.

Then she enters the real world of medical practice. She designs her practice based on what she has seen before and what she can learn from other physicians. Over time she evolves. She learns new skills and incorporates new tools into her practice. She may modify the way patients flow through her office, and care for her hospitalized patients differently as she gains experience. She learns which specialists are the best referral sources. Her care standards are influenced by her colleagues in the community and her specialty organization, and to some extent by the economic incentives she encounters. For the most part, though, the way she cares for patients and organizes her office is the result of how and where she was trained, and the professional socialization she received in the early phases of her career.

The physician is part of a strong culture—the customary beliefs, social forms, and material traits…of (her) group—shared with her physician colleagues. And it is precisely this that makes changing physician behavior so difficult. Think about what must happen to provide the best care possible, why the old and new cultures will clash. A physician has learned to work alone, referring her patient to other physicians if she thinks it is appropriate. The best care possible requires the physician to collaborate with other physicians and the patient (and family, where appropriate) to decide what is best. Instead of being at the top of the medical hierarchy, she is part of a group that may be flat and non-hierarchical. Instead of deciding what gets done for individual patients, she works in partnership with patients and consumers and is accountable with her colleagues for decisions they share. Rather than being compensated for what she alone produces, she may receive income from a pool or a group, divided according to criteria established by the group or system. If in the past she and her physician colleagues shaped the decisions about how the system worked clinically, she now shares those decisions with management, the board and the consumers of the system.

Economic incentives affect the way physicians take care of their patients, of course, but physicians don't do what they do only because of how they are paid. They care for their patients as they've been trained to, as their profession expects them to. Doing so, they believe, is the right and ethical way to practice. They change when they are convinced that care will be better if they do, and when they can imagine themselves practicing that way. Even then they need help to replace deeply ingrained habits and patterns formed over years of professional life. Building an effective process to support this learning, imagining, and replacing old habits with the new ones is essential if you are to transform your organization.

Before we explore how to help physicians through this process, let's remind ourselves how they argue against doing so. Asked to use scientific evidence to make many of their clinical decisions, physicians often complain about "cookbook medicine" even though their own practices reflect cookbooks they internalized in medical school and residency. Greater standardization may be likened to treating patients like widgets in a production line. They may worry about increased legal risk when they must share patient care decisions with other physicians, clinicians, and even the patient herself. Of course financial issues are often mentioned. After practicing in a fee-for-service environment, the changes may seem all loss and no gain, especially for highly paid medical and surgical sub-specialists. If physicians are used to using clinical arguments and threats to get their way with the hospital leaders, it can be upsetting to share that power and influence with non-physicians, and difficult to understand the ethical framework that drives institutional considerations instead of their own clinically based concerns. They complain that the administration doesn't understand what it takes to take care of patients and only worries about the bottom line. They criticize leaders for poor process and for not getting sufficient input to a decision. You get the idea. You probably have your own list.

Arguments like these are predictable no matter how many times you and the physicians join hands in the hot tub and sing "Kumbaya." To create the organizational capabilities you seek requires a thorough understanding of how physicians practice, how they respond to threats, and how they change. Essentially it is one physician at a time. Each physician has to test and experiment in a way that she finds consistent with her commitment to her patients, and that enables her to develop the new habits she will require to care for her patients differently. She needs help to make these shifts. If she can play a role in discovering the alternatives and designing the solutions, then use and improve them with experience, her transition will be smoother. You shortchange this process at your peril.

So what can you do? How can you help your physicians become the agents for change like this? There are several ways to do this. No one of them is sufficient; you need them all. And it takes time and patience.

Common Ground

At the outset you have to establish the common ground you and your physicians share about caring for patients. Most physicians want to do what is best for their patients: heal them, help them get better, and give them the best they know. They don't want them to be harmed, and certainly not die because of preventable errors. They, too, want their patients to be cared for like members of their own family. They probably want the organization to endure and continue to serve the community, and they want to be associated with a system that is respected for its care. If you can agree that you share these things and that this is your common ground, then you have a solid foundation for the next step which is to find who does the best job of providing care this way.

Data and direct observation are key. It helps to review credible data from exemplary organizations that take care of the same kind of patients you do. You can talk to the leaders of these organizations to get access to other information they might have. But your physicians have to see the care firsthand. Take groups from your organization to visit these systems, examine their data, understand how they have achieved their results, and report back what you have seen. Include skeptical physicians who are influential within the medical staff, and make sure they talk to their physician counterparts in the system you are visiting. If a physician can observe what other physicians do, digest the results, look at the data, even talk with the physicians privately, she may reconsider her opposition. And who knows? She could become an advocate for the changes. This hands-on experience is crucial. It expands the common ground you share from an abstract ethical focus to an operational understanding, and helps you move the discussion from whether or not you need to change to how you actually do it.

Information

You also want to present credible information about the performance of the organization and the professionals in it. No matter how carefully you prepare it, though, you can expect challenges. Physicians will argue that their patients are sicker or more difficult. You have to respond to these assertions with more data and more analysis until the arguments stop. Concerns about the integrity of the data must be resolved before you can move on to a discussion of how the organization and each clinician in it is doing, or compare their performance with the best in healthcare. The value of transparency like this is hard to overstate and is worth every cent you have to invest to produce valid and accepted information.

Expect strong resistance at first to any data you produce on individual physician performance. Even if the information is blinded so that only the physician knows which data describes her practice, you are likely to get strong pushback. Visibility and accountability like this are incompatible with traditional views about physician autonomy and professionalism. Once you can show the physicians how to use the data to improve their care, you have begun the data-driven improvement process that is central to delivering the best care possible. Objective information like this is transformative, a powerful tool for moving physicians out of the bunkers they have built to protect their status and maintain their professionalism.

You should eventually make performance information about the organization widely available. From the beginning you should distribute it to your board of directors and your senior team. Eventually it should go to everyone in the organization, and especially to the patients. You may want to go even further. Leaders at Norton HealthCare in Louisville, KY, make their monthly quality report cards available on the web for anyone to see. Whatever you do, be sure to focus on the issues that are most important to patients and consumers: safety, effectiveness, responsiveness, and affordability. Sentinel events, as required by the Joint Commission on Accreditation of Healthcare Organization (JACHO), can be helpful, but you will want to develop even more precise measures of errors and near misses as the baseline for your safety improvement efforts. You want to make sure people understand the evidence-based norms—boundaries—for how specific conditions will be diagnosed and treated in order to track signals that emerge from the "exceptions." You get the idea. The information you collect and discuss reinforces and eventually solidifies the common ground you share with the physicians.

Exposure

As noted, it is important to see firsthand the companies and organizations where exemplary services and products are produced. There is no substitute for this, especially for physicians. It is a conversation changer. When physicians can see what others do and have an opportunity to discuss how that experience applies to their institution, traditional assumptions begin to disintegrate and resistance is muted. From negativity and skepticism, you see a willingness to consider, to try. You may even identify physicians who are prepared to step out front by trying the new approaches. And this is a crucial momentum builder for the changes you seek to make. Strong resistance doesn't disappear with one visit, of course. There are always naysayers, the individuals who refuse to change despite the common ground they share with you, or the information they review, the data they see, or the hands-on experiences. They are too set in their ways, in which case you may need to do some pruning.

Pruning

In a garden you have to prune shoots that are weak or dying to protect the health of the plant and stimulate and shape its growth. You have to do the same with the physicians. Most physicians will respond eventually to persuasion and peer pressures, but a few won't. When a physician is a "flame thrower," a source of trouble and discord in the organization, almost everyone knows it and will watch to see what you will do. You have to act decisively and promptly because these physicians are an organizational cancer; their resistance and behavior can metastasize throughout the organization. Either they change their behavior or they have to go, and the sooner you act, the sooner the organization can get on with what it needs to do. A decision like this sends shock waves through the organization. If physicians perceive that you have acted precipitously or arbitrarily, you will chill the open give and take that you need to move ahead, and damage the common ground you have worked so hard to create. No matter how carefully you act, you can expect to spend a good deal of time reassuring the physicians that this is an exceptional situation rather than the way things will be done going forward. Closing ranks around all but the most egregious performer is normal behavior.

Organization

The advantages of working with an organized group of physicians are significant. It makes your life easier to deal with a limited number of physician-leaders who can represent the larger physician body. You can focus on a smaller group of individuals who, at least theoretically, are in a position to bring their colleagues along. I say "theoretically" because the ability of these leaders to move their colleagues forward depends on their ability to lead and the willingness of the physicians to be led. In a formally organized group, the physicians cede authority to these leaders, and empower them to act on their behalf. Even then, however, the leaders have to work closely with their colleagues to obtain their understanding, support, and involvement before changes can occur.

Groups can be anything from a loose federation of otherwise independent physicians to tightly organized entities like the Permanente Medical Groups or the Mayo Clinic. Whatever form it takes, a formal medical group is no panacea. You trade one set of challenges for another. With independent physicians, you can move faster with some and leave others to catch up. In a formal group, on the other hand, you often cannot move at all until the majority of its members are on board. The voices of the critics can coalesce into formal resistance in an organized group, but are less likely to do so in a network of community physicians. The group, especially one owned by the institution, may focus on work conditions instead of improved patient care. Or the physician leader may not be able to deliver the other physicians, leaving you with few options until she can.

Notwithstanding these concerns, the benefits of having an organized physician group outweigh the disadvantages. To the extent you have any say, the timing for forming a group may be important. It can be easier to launch the change efforts by working with different thought leaders in the physician community in the jujitsu model described earlier. As you gain momentum, you can encourage the formation of a formal physician group if one doesn't exist, or establish a tighter relationship with the group if it does. An important benefit of the formal group is its ability to shape the attitudes of its members, and establish the principles and norms that guide their professional behavior. If the physicians, especially the leaders, are convinced that the changes will enable them to provide better care, then this becomes an important norm for the group that helps persuade and discipline the outliers and engage all the physicians in support of this direction.

Physician groups do not work without excellent leadership, but an all-too-common mistake is to select a respected clinician to do that job. Being a good clinician does not mean the person will be an effective leader. The clinician learns to solve problem through pattern recognition and application of the appropriate precedent and, depending on the specialty, highly developed skills (surgery, interventional radiology, procedures, etc.). She gathers the information, identifies the pattern, provides the accepted care, repeats the cycle as necessary to achieve the best outcome she can, and does the same thing again and again with each successive patient. The challenges a leader faces, in contrast, are often vague, the circumstances ambiguous, and the solutions unclear.

Execution of decisions requires persuasion, cajoling, influencing, patience, and continuous attention to detail as the leader convinces the people who must be involved in these issues. Physicians should be groomed for leadership by giving them opportunities to build these skills in increasingly challenging roles. Without this experience, they are likely to rely on clinical problem solving and relationship skills that are ill suited for most leadership situations. Importantly, it is difficult for someone with few, if any, clinical skills to lead clinicians, although the "professional" physician leader can do so if she is sensitive to the physician culture, and avoids becoming "they,"—part of management by spending considerable time shadowing those who provide the hands-on care.

Ownership

The trend for healthcare systems to buy physician practices is clear. The jury is still out, though, as to whether or not this helps your organization deliver the best care possible. Some physicians join a health system to foster better care coordination and obtain more resources. Others do so to protect themselves and their incomes. Still others sell to the highest bidder, assuming that their lives will be the same in each. A common challenge in owned practices is to maintain productivity once the physicians have joined; typically productivity falls, especially so if the physicians are near the end of their careers. In such circumstances, the energy for making fundamental changes in the culture will be low to non-existent.

Incentives

I will return to the general theme of incentives later (chapter nineteen), but their design for physicians deserves special focus. Any incentives you create must reinforce the vision and values you aspire to instill. Because you want professionals and patients to collaborate in care decisions, the incentives should reward successful patient outcomes that occur as a result. Incentives that reward individual behavior do not do this. Instead they reinforce the traditional physician culture of independence and autonomy that obstructs the very care you wish to deliver.

You should collaborate with your physicians to design the appropriate rewards. Be sure that incentives are flattened across different types of clinical conditions and activities, that they don't reward procedures more than thoughtful diagnosis and treatment, and that they don't pay more for a complex rather than a straightforward patient problem. It may be too big a leap to abandon the fee-for-service (FFS) model entirely, at least at the start. Even if you begin with a hybrid approach, a mix of group and individual incentives, you don't want to lose sight of the larger objective. You can create small, group-focused incentives that reward teams of physicians (as well as other clinicians involved—more on that later) for achieving outcomes of importance to the system as a whole. It doesn't have to be a lot of money. The real value of rewards like these lies in the discussions they generate and the focus they communicate. You can introduce this reward as a supplement to those earned through the traditional fee-for-service system, then increase it over time. How fast you do so depends on where you are in your own system, where the physicians are in their ability to work together to solve common clinical problems, and how rapidly you can push forward in substituting new rewards for the old. Don't be shy, though. You can probably advance more rapidly than you think, especially if the incentive you create is added to, rather than substituted for, what the physicians already earn.

You will want to carve out the incentive pool from the larger revenue pool you control. If you already have physician-incentive pools, an "owned" physician group or a productivity-based rewards pool for example, you can convert them to group rewards. It does not take a lot of money to create the intense focus you seek. At the Northwest Permanente Medical Group, we created a small annual "at risk" compensation pool that represented less than one percent of the total compensation for an individual physician. When it came time to divide up that apparently insignificant pool, it was a dogfight! Bitter complaints arose over the fairness of decisions that produced differences of less than $1,000 per year from one physician to the next. As one colleague observed, physicians are used to being "A" students and view anything less as a failure.

And do not forget the impact of non-financial rewards. These can range from public recognition events for outstanding performance to gift certificates for group dinners, extra time off, or special vacation holidays. You may provide additional resources for teams or groups that meet specific performance targets. Whatever you do, the incentives should always support the new capabilities you are building. Anything that subverts this goal, especially individual incentives of any sort, should be eliminated as rapidly as possible.

You cannot integrate the care you deliver without your physicians. They are the key to delivering care this way. But because of their training and socialization, it is difficult for them to change from an autonomous to collaborative practice. It is imperative, therefore, to establish the common ground and shared values for what you seek to accomplish together. A formal physician organization can help. It is possible to make the changes without one, but the process will proceed more smoothly when the physicians are part of a formal entity that represents their interests, coordinates their contributions, and helps create a new sense of professionalism. The importance of the physician organization exists whether or not physicians are employed by the system. Under any circumstance, you have to be patient, thoughtful, and supportive for physicians to make the transition. Financial incentives help but must reward groups and teams, not individuals, in order to reinforce the collaboration that lies at the heart of the best care possible. And far more than economic rewards are necessary to achieve the fundamental changes you hope to make.

CHAPTER ELEVEN

WORKFORCE

KP began as a commercial organization after World War II when union leaders in the San Francisco Bay Area and the Portland-Vancouver area asked physicians who had cared for their members in the Kaiser ship-yards during the war to continue to do so. They promised to deliver large numbers of union members if the physicians agreed, and they have continued to do so ever since. The workforce at KP is heavily unionized, too (by the mid-nineties, thirty-six unions represented 75 percent of the total workforce through more than fifty separate labor contracts). Although there were tensions, relationships had generally been positive. This changed in the eighties as management and labor became increasingly confrontational. Disputes, work slow-downs, strikes, and difficulties reaching contract agreements occurred frequently. By midway through the 1990s a seemingly endless parade of labor prob-lems required constant attention from leaders on both sides.

Late in 1996, John Sweeney, the president of the AFL-CIO, and I met with a handful of our advisors to see if we could find some way out of the mess we had created. Peter diCicco, a member of John's team, described how the AFL-CIO had collaborated with a handful of man-agement teams in other companies to establish positive, constructive, workforce engagement. He argued that we could do the same, that we too could create an organization in which labor and management, physicians, other clinicians, and support workers joined to take better care of patients and create a more competitive and stable organization. Peter changed the game. Right there. He outlined a roadmap for how we could get there, and John and I agreed to try.

In 1997 KP and the AFL-CIO and their affiliated unions formally approved the labor-management partnership. Three years later 95 percent of our unionized workforce signed a comprehensive national contract that, in the description on the AFL-CIO website at the time, brought "front line caregivers into crucial decisions on staffing levels, quality of care, and business planning through a unique 'partnership' process." When the partner union and management representatives were honored for this achievement, more than five hundred people gathered in a ballroom around small tables spread throughout the room. Working in teams, building trust, and slowly resolving their differences, they had labored for months to hammer out the conditions described in the agreement. Now they sat side by side to hear leaders from the AFL-CIO and KP thank them for what they had accomplished. I remember their faces, their voices, and thinking we finally had the right people working together to help us address the needs of our members. The partnership endures to this day. Throughout the organization at all levels, teams of physicians, nurses, other clinicians, support workers, and union and management representatives join to make things better for patients. It is the way KP does its work.

If the patients vocalize what they need, the people who work in the organization, including the physicians, figure out how to make it happen. They provide the insights and creativity to find the best solutions, and with the right tools improve those solutions with experience. Leaders can't. Neither can consultants or experts. To create this culture of workforce involvement and build the capability to turn that engagement into effective problem solving is challenging. This chapter addresses how you can do it. The term "workforce" refers to the physicians and other clinical professionals and support staff in your system. These more general comments, then, add to those in the previous chapter about engaging your physicians in this effort.

Common Ground

As with physicians, the starting place for workforce engagement is to develop a common ground on which they, you, and the patients stand. Your job as the leader is to provide the first draft of the story about the future that will be revised and rewritten, improved and enriched, in multiple conversations with the workforce, with patients, and with community representatives. This story becomes the shared understanding of what you believe in, what you want to be, and how you will get there. It is your common ground.

Then the magic can happen. It happens when the surgeon and the housekeeper and their fellow workers and patients together figure out how to design and run the pre- and post-operative care system to be as safe, supportive, and efficient as any in the country. Or when they work together to see if they meet their goals and how to improve. It shows in the respect they have for each other's ideas and insights, in the blurring of the differences in their professional status until the outside observer can hardly tell who is the physician, the nurse, the pharmacists, or the housekeeper.

You don't establish a common ground by putting balloons in the atrium, making a few speeches, and hosting a couple of Q&A sessions. It has to define you and the way you work, a central focus of your time and energy—over and over.

Leadership Engagement

To engage the workforce in the care of the patients, you have to engage with them. You have to be where the day-to-day work of the organization takes place, where patients get care, and where the staff helps the clinicians provide the care. You have to know what the people of the organization do, what they think, what they worry about, and what gets in their way. You have to knock down the barriers and obstacles that make their work hard, or you have to explain to them why you can't. You have to do it day in and day out as a consistent, predictable presence.

This is how you learn what is really going on and how you can help make it better. This is how you build the bridges between you as leader and the "real" working people. It is when you model the behaviors and values of the new culture by drawing people out, seeking their advice, honoring their opinions, and the differences among you. It is how you flatten the destructive hierarchies. You do these things with what you say, what you spend your time on, how you engage with those around you, and importantly, by the way you support what others say and do.

Your engagement grows further if you can become involved in people's lives away from work. This is more difficult. By the time we leave work ourselves, we need a break, some distance, and a chance to recover and refuel. We need to protect our health. You can't expect to attend all the events that take place outside of working hours. You have to pick and choose. You have to find what works for you given the organization you lead and your personal life, and you want to do what you do as naturally and comfortably as possible. Here are a few suggestions.

Respect demands that you take part in the mourning for a co-worker or patient who has died. Your presence demonstrates the values that drive you. Other personal events are important too: marriages, graduations, retirements, and illnesses. Any invitation you receive is a gift, an opportunity to establish yet another bridge. The symbolism of your presence reverberates throughout the organization. But this isn't about good politics. The primary motivation is moral. This is the right way to treat each other—the respect that every person, every patient deserves. You want to engage with those around you and value one another, not just in your professional lives but, when appropriate, in your private lives as well. You are in this together and you cannot succeed without one another.

Hardships are another opportunity for people to come together, to provide financial help, food, or clothing, and emotional support. Most of us experienced a profound sense of community in the aftermath of the 9/11 attacks. A similar reaction occurred on a smaller scale when over three hundred Kaiser Permanente people lost their homes in the Oakland

Hills Fire in Oakland, CA, in 1989. They told us about their panic and fear when the fire hit, the confusion about what to take with them in the few minutes they had to evacuate, the shock and sense of loss when they returned to nothing—their homes gone, their possessions burned, many of their memories incinerated. Our people created a support community to provide shelter, financial support, and most importantly emotional support long after the fire had occurred.

Some leaders block daily or weekly time to visit with co-workers where the work is done, where patients are cared for, and support systems operate. This discipline helps them avoid the distractions of other matters. You can also schedule regular meetings with small groups, a breakfast gathering each month, for example, that involves six to eight different people each time from throughout the organization, front-line workers only, no leaders or managers present. The format can be as informal as you like. You want to learn from them and about them, and they about you. You want to demonstrate the values of teamwork and respect, and for them to feel positively enough about the discussion that they share it with their co-workers.

Organizations

The healthcare workforce naturally divides itself into formal and informal groups. Most common are groupings by professional discipline (physicians, nurses, etc.), and by department, service, and location (hospital, outpatient clinics, laboratories, etc.). As described earlier, these can become sources of conflict or divisions within the larger system. But if you work with them, and even formally charter and focus them, they can help you expand workforce involvement and direct their energies to help the people you serve together. For example, you can meet with them on a regular basis to share what is going on and ask their opinions about proposed directions and actions, and to engage them in discussions about the strategies and approaches you and the organization have set out to accomplish. You can ask them to identify patients whose stories would be moving and instructive for the board of directors, your leadership team, or larger audiences throughout the organization. You can ask them to provide written or in-person updates to the board of directors on their contributions to the goals of the organization.

You get the idea. The intent is to make sure they focus their attention on the care delivery transformation rather than the differences among themselves or their disputes with the organization or its leaders. To do this, you have to be consistent in your relationships, using these and other tools to involve them. You may find that mini-organizations or groups are of little consequence in your setting, that they aren't worth the effort required. Whatever your circumstances, you should be alert to their emergence, especially if they start to resist the changes and worry more about protecting their own territory than the well-being of the larger organization.

Unions

If you have unions in your system, you know that they bring their own agendas to the relationship with the organization. We know what happens when these relationships go bad, when groups within the workforce are at odds with the goals of the organization. These confrontations make it difficult, if not impossible, to achieve your objectives in the service of the patient and patient care. You have to find an alternative to this destructive cycle of contention, stalemate, and resolution. Few examples exist in- or outside healthcare in the US. Toughness with labor is equated with good leadership; conflicts between labor and management are expected. An undercurrent of suspicion infects the organization and further divides workers and leaders. Our divisive political rhetoric reflects this too—a hatred of unions on the one hand, and support for them on the other. The labor-management partnership at Kaiser Permanente is a positive alternative.

Tensions still exist, of course. Trust can be fragile, actions misinterpreted. Participants struggle to balance the interests of union members with those of the workforce and organization. But the partnership has shown that it is possible to work through these issues, and strengthen the organization by deepening the engagement of the workforce as a result. The partnership has contributed to the continued improvement of care for patients throughout the system. As hokey as it might sound, it has created a sense of a family, directed toward the same goals, committed to one another, respecting each other, and dealing constructively with the inevitable internal squabbles that arise.

Interest Groups

Another way to engage the workforce is through formally chartered interest groups. These are usually organized around ethnicity and sexual orientation. A number of companies, for example, have established organizations of African American, Latino, Asian, and Gay, Lesbian, Bi-Sexual, Transgender (GLBT) employees. You don't want them to have to lobby for their "rights," as this inevitably leads to tensions throughout the organization and is an impediment for the changes. Instead you want to charter them to:

- Help you, the leadership, and the system understand how patients from different ethnic or personal backgrounds are cared for now.

- Understand the market segments you are trying to reach, and the marketing and sales issues you must address to reach these specific segments,

- Understand the specific relationship issues a particular ethnic or personal interest group faces as employees of the system, and help develop programs to educate the workforce as appropriate,

- Identify and recruit people into the system, including suggesting potential members for the board of directors, and

- Organize events that bring the members together to create a sense of community.

To realize these benefits and avoid the detrimental behaviors that can sometimes arise, you should charter the organizations formally and provide at least token financial support for their work. The charter specifies the purposes of the group and establishes a formal system for setting and reviewing long term goals and objectives that fit within the larger context of the system. The money required to support their work is usually small in absolute terms, and especially so when compared to the potential benefits these organizations bring if organized and directed properly.

Story Telling

Stories are the most powerful tool for bringing people together. They help us learn and remember and find our shared humanity. What stories are helpful to the transformation like this one? All of them! Stories about patients and stories told by the patients and their families. Stories about the care that employees or their family have received from the system. Stories about hardships, volunteer work, hobbies, and interests outside of work. It doesn't matter. What matters is the story, the act of telling it, the storyteller and the audience, the sharing. The more often you do this—the more aspects of people's lives are shared this way—the stronger the bonds you build among you.

Certain stories have special impact. Those about the care patients receive, the needs they have when they are sick or injured, and the challenges they face in getting care are the most powerful. When a patient tells his story, it can really affect us. We feel the pain or the fear, the frustrations, and even the rage when things have gone badly. We share the sense of loss and profound sadness, or the joy of return to good health. Although stories about taking care of patients aren't as powerful, they are important too. What's it like to be a nurse on the night shift when a patient has a cardiac arrest? What's it like to work with an insulting physician or a disagreeable co-worker? What's it like to work a twelve-hour shift at the hospital, come home to feed the kids, then head out to night school to pursue the degree that may give you a chance at higher wages?

Stories that involve the lives of fellow workers outside of healthcare are also valuable, their volunteer work or community service, for example. These, too, can help people see each other in a different light. The beauty of stories is that they can be told about many subjects in so many ways. A first person story is best. Surveys, statistics, studies, and science obscure the realities of what it means to be sick and scared, or hurt or frustrated, injured or ignored by the very people the patient relies on for help. But when patients tell their stories in their own words, they open our eyes and touch the emotions we share.

The availability of other communications tools, such as video magazines, Facebook, Twitter, blogs, etc., expands the opportunities to tell individual stories. You have to use them with care though. There can be too much information, too many stories, so many in fact that people become numb and indifferent. As in so many other aspects of leadership, you have to find the balance that works for your situation. But even when people hear stories on the same subject again and again, it is hard to ignore a patient or co-worker who stands in front of them, looks them in the eye, and challenges them to understand and care. Real stories told by real people rarely get old.

A final consideration is the target audience. Who needs to hear these stories, especially those from patients? The answer is simple: everyone. This is the most powerful tool you have to shape the culture of your organization. Physicians, the board of directors, the senior leadership team, the larger leadership group, and the workforce itself need to be immersed in these stories to escape the traps of their own backgrounds, professions, their formal fiduciary responsibilities, and their busy lives. To compel them to change, to become patient-centric, they need to hear what happens to the people they care for, what it's like to be these people, what it is about the care that makes their lives better or more difficult. Properly designing changes in care requires data, good information, careful analysis, and wide input from different perspectives. Being compelled to change long-standing practices requires something more powerful—the stories told by real people about their lives.

Fun

Award ceremonies, recognition systems, games and contests, silly competitions—there are many ways to bring fun, even joy, to the workplace.

You have to work at it, though, because what we do in healthcare is so serious. Our satisfaction comes from being professional, being excellent, and bringing relief. Building a sense of community requires more, however, and that's where fun comes in.

Weave award ceremonies and recognition systems into the fabric of your organization. You might want to adapt one or more of the awards that KP gives into your own institution:

- **Annual Awards for Quality:** To promote teamwork and healthy competition, nominate care teams to receive an annual award for patient quality. The criteria should focus on multi-disciplinary teamwork and measured impact on quality outcomes for patients. Invite the awardees to an annual dinner/awards ceremony attended by most of the senior leaders, your board of directors, and your Union partners if you have them. Have the chair of the board's Quality Committee present the award. Make sure considerable publicity is provided to the winning teams throughout the organization.

- **Annual Awards for Patient Safety:** Similar to the quality awards, recognize teams of caregivers for significant contributions to improved patient safety. Select the winners based on their efforts to improve safety or adapt a safety innovation from either another part of the organization or from outside. The patient safety awards, then, should encourage both innovation and diffusion.

- **Annual Awards for Community Service:** Here the focus is on volunteering in the community. You might want to acknowledge a group of employees who have made a particular contribution. You might also want to recognize individual efforts. Provide each winner with a financial contribution from the Program to the volunteer project they have supported.

In addition to awards like these, you can hold annual conferences on quality, safety, community service, as well as workforce diversity, to name several. These should reinforce the vision and priorities of the organization, and highlight the work people do every day. Presentations should be made by the people of the organization in small groups, work groups, and gatherings of all the attendees. Award winners can be announced in conjunction with these gatherings.

And of course, there should be an opportunity for real fun, for laughing, and sharing beyond the workplace: picnics and races, special food dishes, Halloween costume contests, etc. You are limited only by your imagination when it comes to bringing people together this way. You want to involve the physicians if you can. Physicians tend to be a serious lot, intent on their individual interests when they aren't taking care of their patients. Being silly may be considered unprofessional. But even if the physicians choose not to take part, these activities are worth doing. They help reduce the distances among the people of the organization and between leaders and the workforce. And, who knows? Perhaps the physicians will see what they're missing and join in at some point!

Retreats and Other Strategic Gatherings

Planned and executed well, formal gatherings away from the worksite also foster cohesion and a common sense of purpose. These can be large or small, held in modest settings, and not cost an arm and a leg. They bring people together to consider long-term matters, or to address issues that are difficult to resolve in the course of daily work. Planned well, they reinforce the sense of community, and address challenging questions of importance to the organization. They should not be loosely organized experiences that you hope will pay dividends at some point in the future. You have to pay attention to the subjects you will consider: two or three are better than five or six. Meetings like these should be part of the annual calendar so that those involved know they will happen and when. You might bill the retreat as the start of or part of an annual planning cycle. Or you can use it to consider issues that require more time and reflection than is possible during regular working hours. You can add off-site events as needed throughout the year, but be careful not to overuse them. You don't want to use them to put off decisions that should be made on the spot.

Other Ideas

Some organizations use a formal suggestion system to encourage people to offer their ideas for improving the care in the system. These can be anonymous or attributed; they can be in writing or e-mail; they can be recognized if used and even rewarded with cash or other in-kind awards (a gift certificate, etc.). Surveys are useful tools to determine how much employees understand about the values, directions, and common ground you wish to build into the entire workforce. They can help assess the level of commitment to these ideals, as well as the engagement people have with making things better. You also can use them to determine how well leaders are working with people on the front lines. The most useful are short and focused, reinforced by feedback from the leaders, acted upon when appropriate, and not done frequently.

You may want to write a CEO newsletter, distributed by mail, e-mail, Twitter, or whatever works for you. George Halvorson, the recently retired CEO of Kaiser Foundation Health Plan and Hospitals, wrote a weekly e-mail letter to everyone in the organization for more than a decade. The subject you choose should reflect what's important to you and to the state of your organization. Whatever its focus, it should reinforce your quality agenda. It's also a good way to build bridges throughout the organization, and an excellent complement to the direct interactions you have as you work side by side with your co-workers.

Your partnership with the workforce is yet another lever for transforming your organization. You cannot succeed without the ideas and expertise, the energy and passion of those who care for patients, or the support of those who provide the care. It all starts with you. Before you can expect the workforce to be engaged in the values and purpose of the system, you have to engage with them as their leader, and together build a shared sense of values and purpose and commitment to one another. The tools at your disposal are limited only by your imagination. They range from efforts to shape the agendas and work of the formal and informal mini-organizations that exist within any larger system; to using stories, especially those of patients, to shape the culture and its values; to using recognition programs to encourage sharing and innovation and results. They include activities that focus on fun and on building connections that complement what occurs at the worksite. All have a single purpose: to create and maintain a community of co-workers who share the goal of creating the new culture and new capabilities that enable them to provide the best care possible to each patient.

CHAPTER TWELVE

COMPACTS

A compact[5] is an explicit agreement between two parties. Like vows in the marriage ceremony, it symbolizes and documents the joining of parties in partnership. Born of mutual dependence, it is an explicit promise to collaborate and cooperate. It describes the shared purposes and values, and the responsibilities each has to the other, often in language that can be quite precise in an effort to achieve clarity and preclude misunderstandings or misapprehensions. It is not a contract, however. A contract is a legally binding document that details the responsibilities of each party, the process for resolving differences and contingencies, and, typically, the economic rights and penalties. The compact is not necessarily legally binding and is usually silent on dispute resolution and issues of restitution and damages.

The conversations that lead to a final written compact are where the understandings and commitments are explored, disagreements are surfaced, and words and phrases are revised until they communicate a common understanding. It is when the important "what-if" and "do-you-mean" issues appear. The process of arriving at a written agreement—

---

[5] I am indebted to Gary Kaplan, MD, the chairman and CEO of Virginia Mason Health System, for introducing me to this term.

the discussions, the writing, rewriting, and the editing—is almost as valuable as the final written agreement itself. This exploration and the resulting written agreement is important to the transformation of your organization. It is particularly helpful for the physicians to know what to expect from you during this transition, just as you want clarity from them about their commitments to you. You may wish to create a compact between you and your board of directors. You can do the same with different professional groups or even interest groups (see chapter eleven). Developed and finalized this way, the compact becomes the framework for the way you work together to transform the organization. Ideally it endures; it shouldn't need frequent revisions, though you will benefit by revisiting it regularly together to be sure you remain on track with its intent.

With this in hand, the physicians, for example, can be more precise about how they manage themselves, and how they recruit new physicians. The compact lays out the expectations, both for them as physicians, and from the larger organization. This clarity helps physicians who are being recruited to decide whether or not they wish to live with the agreement and in this environment. The same is true for managers and leaders, and for board members too. They learn in advance what the expectations are, what the agreement is, and whether or not they want to embrace them. When they join, they do so with their eyes wide open.

A written compact like this can be especially useful when conflicts or disagreements arise. Rather than ignore the issues or resolve them through a formal dispute resolution process, you can revisit the agreement together, discuss yet again the commitments you have made to one another, judge the disagreement in that context, and work together to resolve the matter. This reinforces your mutual interdependence and your shared purpose, and allows you to explore once again what your partnership means and how you can achieve what you both envision.

It isn't all sweetness and light, though. Compacts can't solve everything. But it is far better than the traditional contract approach because it is based on mutual trust and explicit promises rather than legal obligations. Two examples illustrate how these work.

As described in the introduction, Kaiser Permanente is made up of two interlocking not-for-profit entities, Kaiser Foundation Health Plan and

Kaiser Foundation Hospitals (KFHP/H) and the independent Permanente Medical Groups (PMGs). An umbrella entity, the Permanente Federation, represents the Medical Groups in specific areas defined in a master agreement among the parties. With this confusing, multi-level, geographically dispersed organization, imagine how hard it can be to reach agreements. Imagine too the conflicts that arise between the interests of physicians and their medical group, and the interests of the Health Plan and Hospitals organization. How does it work as well as it does?

It almost didn't. In the mid-1950s the organization, then much smaller and less complex, nearly fell apart because of continuing disagreements between the physician groups and the Health Plan/Hospitals organization, and among the physician groups themselves. After long and difficult discussions, an agreement was reached that clarified the responsibilities and commitments of the parties. The written document, called the Tahoe Agreement because it was finalized in 1955 at the vacation home of Henry Kaiser at Lake Tahoe, became the glue for the organization for forty years. It provided the framework needed to work together, serve each other's interests, resolve concerns about territory, and maintain the community of interest that lies at the heart of this partnership-based organization.

By the mid-1990s the world had changed and the internal dynamics of the organization had shifted too. Instead of five medical groups, there were twelve. Instead of a west-coast-centric organization, the regions covered eighteen states and Washington, DC. Instead of one million members the organization served eight million. Efforts to redefine the organization and the relationships to accommodate these realities led to escalating conflicts. The original agreement was invoked time and time again, but eventually the parties realized that it was no longer up to the task. A new agreement was required. Following intense work over many months, the new agreement was signed in a formal ceremony. It reaffirmed the core principles that had guided the organization for so long: partnership and mutuality, and the exclusive commitment the physician groups and the KFHP/H organization made to one other.

The details of these two agreements are fascinating, especially to someone who lived with them. But what is most relevant here is that they are one kind of compact. The first lasted forty years; the second is still in effect after fifteen years. They are living agreements that have been central to how the parties work together, and for establishing the trust that enables the organization to make decisions and resolve internal conflicts. While both contain contract-like language, this is a reflection of the many parties involved, and the need to create promises that are as explicit and clear as possible. The agreements are short on philosophy except for what matters: the partnership, the commitment to one another, and the agreement to do things for each other and on behalf of the entire organization.

Virginia Mason leaders have used a different compact to describe the commitments between the leadership of the organization and its physician group. Theirs is short, simple, and direct; it is written in clear, declarative, unambiguous language. Its roots are firmly embedded in the realities of Virginia Mason and the relationship, not in ambiguous clouds of hopes and dreams. Its origins, its shaping, and its words give it considerable power. The impact of this process, as well as the value of the agreement in practice, led the board of directors to create a compact between themselves and the organization that makes explicit the same promises to one another.

According to the dictionary, the term "compact" means a joining or compressing, implying a narrowing of the distances that separate. The word "covenant," especially in Biblical reference, refers to promises— commitments that are deep and philosophical. The Tahoe Agreements are compacts and covenants at once; they narrow the distances among the parties, compressing and joining them in mutual purpose, while articulating profoundly held promises about how they work together and support one another. The Virginia Mason compacts are the same. In both examples, the language and the process to get to that language brought into the open what is too often left unstated in healthcare about what to expect and how to work with one another. Searching for the words to describe the promise and the mutual obligations deepened the commitment and bonds the parties more tightly.

The partnerships described in part two require collaboration and shared work to achieve your common purpose. You cannot get there any other way. Think about taking this one step further. Think of the benefit of agreeing explicitly to how this will happen, what you promise to do for and with one another. Imagine how helpful it is to have a common path through the conflicts, past the obstacles, and over the barriers that lie ahead. Think about the value of returning to it together as a team again and again over the years: refining it as you need to, clarifying what it means, and working through your disagreements. A compact helps avoid the worst possible outcome for you and for your organization: when disagreements and conflicts lead each party to retreat into its space, lick its wounds, and look for ways to get even.

PART THREE

SYSTEMS

Docking a large ship in a narrow waterway requires a carefully choreo-
graphed dance among the captain, the crew, the tugboats, and the people
at the dock in which the captain's skills and experience join those of the
people around him. You must do the same in healthcare, except you will
need a more comprehensive and enduring approach to achieve your goal.
Seven core systems enable you to do this. Each is powerful, but only when
joined together in a robust operating discipline do they provide the force
you need to move your organization in the direction you have chosen.

The first of these is the system of language: the words, actions, and
symbols you use to build and maintain common purpose. The second is
the learning system you establish that makes the search for ever-better
care the obsession of the organization. The third system is directed to
transparency, illuminating decisions, performance, and progress for all
to see. Fourth is innovation, intended to introduce a steady stream of
new ways to provide care in order to keep the organization fresh,
looking outward, and watching what others do. Next is the system you
use to gather, store, move, and use the information needed to care for
patients, manage the organization, and lead its transformation. Sixth is
the system you use to prod the organization towards the future you
have chosen. The final system deals with accountability and its com-
panions—compensation and rewards.

Together these seven systems, described in chapters thirteen through nineteen, create the context, the soul, the meaning for what the organization provides, and how it operates. They help you shape the organization in a continuous molding, prodding, and pushing, that river-like, finds new channels for its flow. In chapter twenty, we explore the operating discipline that brings together your leadership, your partners, and your systems into a coherent whole.

CHAPTER THIRTEEN

LANGUAGE

Early one morning I took the first flight from the Bay Area to San Diego to deliver the opening speech to a large gathering of quality leaders from around the Program. My wife and I had attended a Rolling Stones concert the night before. I was sleep deprived and my ears were still ringing as I approached the stage to speak. Just before I started up the stairs, a physician colleague grabbed my arm and whispered, "For God's sake, don't give another one of your doom-and-gloom talks!" Of course that was what I had planned, so by the time I reached the microphone, I had no idea what to say. I winged it instead.

My Mick Jagger moonwalk imitation was a bust, but the audience relaxed and laughed at my obvious lack of skills. Then I described the day my grandmother asked me to end her life. She'd moved to a nursing home in the late stages of a long and debilitating battle with a rare cancer. I spoke about losing someone I loved and what it meant as a physician to be faced with an ethical dilemma like this. I talked about the promise we make as providers to do no harm and to work on behalf of our patients, our members, and our communities. And that was it. No doom and gloom. No statistics. Just a personal story preceded by a half-baked joke at my expense.

People in the audience that day still laugh about my lousy moonwalk and tell me how deeply touched they were by the story of my grandmother, how it made them think about why they worked in healthcare, and how they've dealt with similar situations. They remember the talk even though it happened more than fifteen years ago. I gave hundreds of doom-and-gloom talks as CEO, and not one person has told me she remembered a word I said in those presentations.

Every word you use, phrase you create, story you tell, argument you make, explanation you give, communication you send, action you take—virtually everything you do as the leader—tells the people around you who you are. You are defined through impressions collected over time, filtered through the lenses of others. You are more than that, of course, but no matter what you do, your language shapes the perceptions that people form of you as their leader. Language really matters, especially so as you articulate the direction the organization has chosen to take. It matters as you describe how you will carry out the journey, what you will and won't do, what behaviors you will and won't allow, and will and won't reward. You must use it well to be able to convey what you think is important, what motivates you. To create great followers—people who are committed and creative, who spend their time finding better ways to serve the patients and customers of the institution—you must be a great leader. And to be a great leader requires you to master the language of leadership.

Words and phrases are the first building block. Some are louder than others and drown out those they accompany. For example healthcare leaders often describe their mission as delivering "quality, affordable care," or words to this effect. "Affordable" is an especially loud word. Many physicians and other clinicians, and patients as well, often think "affordable" means "cheap" and the quality of patient care must be compromised to achieve it. Or consider the phrase "patient-centric care." It's an overused phrase that has lost its meaning. And when paired with a loud word like "affordability," or "cost-effectiveness," or "efficiency" in healthcare, its importance is lost altogether.

Combining quality, safety, patient experience, and affordability and efficiency in the description of your mission confuses the argument for focusing on superior quality in the first place. You want to deliver the best-known care to patients. Period. Everything else follows.

We often use too many words and try to make so many points the meaning is lost. Whether speaking or writing, it is important to be spare, clear, and unambiguous. Use action words. Be declarative. Don't complicate. Make sure your audience can hear the important words. Don't clutter your messages with too many ideas. Don't confuse your followers with Christmas tree explanations, in which every idea and argument you can think of is hung like an ornament to be sure you say it all. You want to guide and teach, to help people focus on what is important. You don't have to impress them with how much you know. They will stop listening after the first few words if you do; instead of "wise," they will think "boring" the next time you open your mouth.

As you've heard time and time again in this book, stories are the best way to communicate what is important. People remember them because good ones touch their memories, experiences, empathy, fears, joys, and passions. A rich scientific literature supports this observation. So do centuries of human communications. YouTube is nothing more than a collection of video stories. Patient stories about their experiences are the most powerful of all, especially when patients or family members tell them. You can use their stories to illustrate the points you want to make, but you have to be careful. Chances are someone in the organization knows the story better than you do, so if you aren't accurate or exaggerate in some way, co-workers will know right away. Your stories must be clear and short; no one wants to listen to you tell a complicated story, especially in the groups or larger gatherings in which you are at the podium. You can also sound phony, like the politician citing Joe the Plumber down the street. You want to use patient stories wisely if you tell them. Better still, let the patients tell their stories themselves.

There are many other ways to communicate with the organization. Most common are meetings, gatherings, groups, or the on-the-floor visits.

Whenever you can, you need to look people in the eye, see how they respond, hear their questions, and read their body language. You can test your language this way too, trying different stories, making your points differently, using alternate words, always seeking a more powerful way to convey what is important to you. You can also write, or, if you don't write well, you can find someone in your organization to write for you. Everything you send out should go through a filter, a trusted reader or two who makes sure your messages are clear and simple and consistent with what you've said before.

Your actions are part of the language of leadership too: what you do, where you spend your time, how you talk with people, what decisions you make, and how you talk about those decisions. Critically important is how you spend your time. If you say patients are important, your people will believe you only if you regularly spend time with real patients. If you visit the workplaces but use your time to tell everyone what they need to do, your message of inclusion and respect will be lost. If you punish someone for making a mistake, the message you send is that specific results are more important than learning why the mistake occurred and how to prevent it in the future. Actions matter. They *do* speak louder than your words. And when your actions reinforce your words, you use the most powerful leadership language of all.

Whatever your language, consistency is critical. Most organizations do not do well with ambiguity or uncertainty. Starting something without following through fosters cynicism and deepens resistance. If you plan to hold a regular meeting with the organization, do it. If you plan to visit people at work, do it regularly, not whenever you can squeeze it in. If you have an opportunity to make a point on the spot, don't wait.

Most of us struggle to be consistent. There are too many distractions. We are pulled in many directions each day. But as leaders, we not only communicate by what we do and say, but especially by what we do all the time, by what others can "set their watches by" in our schedule. People look for reasons to not change. Most would prefer to do what they've always done. Your lack of follow-through is often reason enough.

If you're not serious enough to do the things you say are important, the people won't be serious about them either. Worse, they make up stories to explain what you've failed to do; they give your inconsistency a twist that suits their interests.

And then there are the symbolic acts of leadership that assume almost iconic importance in defining you, and in conveying your expectations and values. The first time I met with the large leadership group of Kaiser Permanente as their CEO designate, my predecessor, Jim Vohs, introduced me by putting his arm around my shoulder when we entered the room. His simple message—there is continuity here.

Props help too. To show the way their partnership worked in their Kaiser Permanente region, the medical director and regional manager always held up a yardstick, pointed to the first and last inches on it to emphasize the few things they did separately, then to the remaining thirty-four inches to represent the decisions they made together.

Throughout your leadership journey, you walk a fine line. You don't want to be so aloof that people have little first-hand knowledge on which to create their stories about you; they fill the void with rumors and partial truths. But you also don't want to be so accessible that you have a hard time conveying the tough messages, or making the difficult changes that are the leader's responsibility. You can't be "one of the boys" and lead effectively. Nor can you be so distant and unknown that you have few, if any, connections with your followers. You can't lead from the mountaintop and you can't lead when you are one of the gang. You have to strike a balance.

With this as background, here are a number of ways to use language to move your institution toward the best care possible:

Make Quality the Centerpiece

Quality defines what you are reaching for: the best-known care for your patients delivered to meet their needs, every time. You must not drown out this core message by adding louder words around it: cost-effective care, affordable care, efficient care. Be simple and direct and unambiguous; quality is the focus. You cannot say it often enough: if everyone does the right things for your patients, everything else will follow. Convey your confidence in the model and methods you've chosen to deliver quality. Convey too that your focus on quality will deliver the savings—the strong bottom line you must have to remain in business, to compete. And never cut staff or services to save costs. These actions smother your quality message and derail the very efforts that are central to your future.

Attend and Participate in the Orientations of New Employees

Try never to miss an orientation, and always lead the presentations about the mission, methods, and values that the organization believes in. Use a story or two to make your points. Have a patient make the point too if you can arrange it. Be clear about what you expect, and make it personal. Let your passion show. Ask for questions, and respond candidly. Don't be afraid to disagree or challenge. And if you see someone at the orientation who clearly doesn't fit it, don't hesitate to speak to her in private to ask her to leave before she can infect those around her.

Schedule Rounds to the Places Where People Work

Management by walking around works. To make it useful, you need to organize it properly and do it frequently enough to matter. Block it into your annual calendar at the beginning of the year and don't deviate except in an emergency. Always take the time to explain why you were unable to meet this commitment if you have to cancel. Separate presentation visits from more informal information-gathering and relationship-building visits. Do both. Presentation visits should be organized as joint working sessions in which you, your senior team, relevant managers, and the people on the line review and discuss the work, and make suggestions and take actions to enable the work to move forward. Stay away from show and tell; make it more real, focused, and purposeful.

For the relationship-building visits, you want to learn what's going on, what's preventing people from doing their work, what frustrates them or makes them happy, and what they are committed to and what they are not. It's a chance to ask questions, and to teach by illustrating a relationship to the larger organizational purpose or values. You should listen far more than you talk; a good rule of thumb is that others speak more than 70 percent of the time, and you less than 30 percent when you are together in these kinds of gatherings.

Write a Regular Column or Newsletter

As mentioned earlier, this is a particularly effective tool when the organization is large and it is hard to reach everyone in person. It also helps you simplify and reinforce your messages about care quality. And it is flexible. You can tell short stories. You also can recognize any outstanding work that people have done to further the agenda. Do it regularly enough that people look for it, and make it short enough that busy people will read it. Use language that communicates with the most educated and the high school dropout. If you have workers for whom English is a second language, publish a translation in their first language.

Join a Team, Class, or Community Project Where Fellow Workers are Involved

It is valuable to find a non-work-related activity that can bring you together with employees and professionals from your organization. The more informal and "fun" the better. You want to share time with your employees away from work, and give them a closer glimpse of who you are. Choose something that you will commit to and want to do. If you can involve your own family, even better. Church activities, volunteer work, a specific community project like Habitat for Humanity, fund-raising walks, for example, are ways to interact away from the demands of work and do good at the same time.

This is an eloquent way to demonstrate your shared values. Your commitment of time and energy away from the workplace is visible and noticed. You can't fake it though. You can't show up once and then never appear again. You can't arrive and fail to participate. Just as your actions are watched at work, they are observed away from work as well.

Attend Patient and Employee Funerals and Special Events

As mentioned in chapter eleven, attend the funeral of every patient and employee if it is open, and try to attend funerals, weddings, and special events to which you are invited by an employee or patient: Early in our marriage, my wife made an emergency visit to the East Coast to see her ailing father. When he passed away, she asked me to come to the funeral despite the fact that we were living on a shoestring at the time. I hemmed and hawed until a friend living with us at the time tore into me, saying, "What is more important than the funeral of someone you care about?" I had lost sight of what mattered.

Our lives are a complex tapestry of work, family, hobbies, special events, heartbreak, and individual achievements. This shapes us; it feeds or compromises our spirits; and it affects our ability to engage in our work. We cannot disentangle our work from our lives. In the poem "Two Tramps in Mud Time," Robert Frost reminds us "...work is play for mortal stakes." As the leader of the organization, it is important to show people that you know this by taking the time to attend the funeral of an employee, or responding to an invitation to join the funeral of a family member, a wedding, or a special event. You show that every individual is important enough for you to be there both on your own and as the leader of the organization with which the individual was associated. You aren't looking for praise or thanks, nor is this in your job description. It is simply what you expect of yourself as a leader and human being.

What comes of this in terms of the wider perceptions will happen with or without your help. You do need to be aware, however, that you never just represent yourself; you are always a symbol, always the leader. What you say and do, the manners and respect and kindness you show, the time you spend, will be interpreted by those you lead, regardless of the occasion.

Seek Opportunities to Show Your Passion about the Care Patients Receive in Your Organization

We learn early in our professional lives to "control" our emotions. Physicians, for example, are taught Osler's principle of "equanimitas"—to be calm and objective. We're almost afraid of some emotions: too much joy, too much anger, too much sadness. Who cries when a patient dies? Who rages when a patient is injured because of an error? Who is thrilled by an improvement that benefits a particular patient? Who laughs unselfconsciously at the many ridiculous things we do and say in the course of a day? When do we allow ourselves the full range of our humanity? Why do we button down our emotions as healthcare professionals?

During a meeting I attended, the chairman of the board of Children's Hospital in Cincinnati described his outrage when he learned about a preventable error that caused injury or death to a child in the hospital. He became so upset he couldn't sleep. It was worse than being kicked in the gut. He sought other board members who responded the same way. The chief of Anesthesiology in the Colorado Permanente Medical Group once nearly killed a patient on the operating table by injecting the wrong drug. When he told the family what had happened, he cried. And they comforted him, and thanked him for telling them the truth.

Why not? What's wrong with that? What's wrong with showing joy when a team of caregivers and a patient improve care by working together and designing a new way to do things? What's wrong with showing anger, even losing your cool sometimes, in the most egregious situations? If your emotions are real, not manufactured to make a point, they convey important messages to those around you. People respond to your emotions more strongly than to the words you use.

I've never understood the notion of playing it cool, of not showing emotions, as if doing so weakens you, lessens you as a leader. It doesn't make sense. The first task of preparing to lead is to find your moral core, the fire in your belly that drives you, the beacon that lights the way for you. It doesn't have to be out there for everyone to see; it doesn't have to show all the time or even very often. You have to do it in a way that is consistent with who you are as a person. However you show it, there is no reason to hide it behind a veneer of objectivity and emotional distance. You want people to know what is important to you, and you cannot communicate this with words alone. When your responses communicate your values and your passions, the messages are loud and consequential. People remember.

Conduct Regular Language Audits

You will develop a sense of how well you communicate with the people of the organization. Consciously or unconsciously, you'll make course corrections as you move ahead. To really understand, though, you need the help of more objective observers. The best person for this is someone in the organization who has a rich network and can talk openly with you, a truth-teller you can count on to share her perceptions, whatever they are. If you don't have someone like this, you can hire an outside expert to conduct a formal assessment. You will be best served by using both: an inside person with whom you meet regularly and an outsider to conduct periodic formal audits of your performance. You want them to help you answer several important questions. Are people hearing what you want to convey? How do they perceive you as their leader? Can they see and feel your passion? Do they know what is important to you?

Hire a Communications Consultant to Help You with Spoken and Written Communications

It is hard for most people to be concise and use simple, declarative language. A good communications consultant can help you prepare for speeches and meetings by getting rid of all but the key two or three points, by reshaping your language to be more accessible, and by remaking your sentences to be declarative and action-based. She can help you get rid of the caveats, the tangents, and the tedious explanations, and only use words and rhythms that convey your passion and beliefs.

In college we were required to attend two fifteen-minute non-religious chapel gatherings each week first thing in the morning. The speaker had ten to twelve minutes to discuss his subject. Some were coherent and memorable, others were forgotten the minute we left the building. We grew to appreciate how difficult it was to reduce a message to its essence, to the few critical points described in pristine, memorable language. The language of leadership is like that. Used well, it reinforces the vision and values of your organization. Used poorly, it leads to misunderstandings, even skepticism, and obscures the core vision and values that will define your future.

Your language creates the context, and the stories about what you want to happen and about you as the leader. It is imperative to keep your messages clean, simple, straightforward, and memorable. Words and actions matter. It takes work, and sometimes help from others, to craft the right ones into the compelling stories that move an organization ahead. None of this can be done on the fly. Language is too important to be left to chance.

CHAPTER FOURTEEN

LEARNING

Jack Welch, the former chairman and CEO of General Electric, was a tough, performance-obsessed leader. He also invested heavily in learning. I once spent a day with him to explore the lessons he had learned as he transformed GE. He was warm, expansive, funny, profane, and insightful. Some of his observations were hard to translate to our situation, but many were quite relevant. One of the most interesting was how Welch and his team created the environment to support and invested in continuous learning. One story I've heard several times in different settings is illustrative:

A young executive made a strategic bet that resulted in a loss for his division. By the time he met with Welch, he was a nervous wreck. Welch noted his shaking hands and uncontrollable sweating and asked what was wrong. The executive explained that he expected to be fired for losing so much money. "Fire you!" Welch reportedly yelled. "Why would I fire you when we just spent $20 million on your education?"

To provide the best care possible requires an unceasing quest to find better ways to deliver care. It is an obsession. Learning like this must be planned. It doesn't happen by chance. You have to create the learning environment, design the learning system for your organization, and then consistently reinforce the importance of learning with your words and actions.

You begin with language and values: how you talk about inquiry and experimentation; the importance you place on discovering new ways to care for patients; and the way you demonstrate your fascination with what others do outside of your organization, and even outside of healthcare. It includes how you support people when they try and fail, but learn from their mistakes; and the help you give your workforce to learn from each other and use good ideas wherever they find them. It is the way your leadership team works: constructively criticizing, rarely punishing, consistently supporting and encouraging, and searching for new solutions. It is the systems you build to deliver information needed for learning and improving. What you create, then, is a culture that includes a system and metrics to reinforce the drive to get better. This is not learning for its own sake, but a relentless focus on providing the best care for your patients.

On a wall outside an Agilent Technologies manufacturing production line in Singapore were charts that plotted a rapid improvement in product reliability (shown as reduced defect rates) over a six-week period and a similar drop in the cost per unit produced in that same timeframe. The line manager explained that he and his team looked at every instance of performance that fell outside the planned tolerances to determine why, then improved. They did this again and again until they reached their desired target of 3.4 defects for every million units produced (a six sigma level of reliability). After that, they introduced innovations that produced even higher performance and made the product even more reliable to produce.

By establishing tolerance limits and focusing on those events outside them, the managers made rapid and dramatic improvements in the quality of their product. This is the way most learning takes place in a production environment. Stripped of its mysteries, healthcare is a production environment, and we can learn this way too. You measure what you do, design an improved solution, implement it, and measure again in a continuous loop. You focus your efforts where they will pay off. You cannot respond to everything, every whim, everyone's pet bias. You have to know when things work as planned and when they don't to determine how to get better.

There is variation in almost everything we do, including our work. The question is how to know when variation exceeds what we expect, how we know what to investigate to find out if something might be wrong. For this you need signals that distinguish unexpected from routine variation in the care you provide. How? To begin, you must establish what is "expected" or "acceptable." This applies to how physicians care for a patient with moderate to severe asthma. It applies as well to how a patient moves through admission to discharge for a knee replacement or diagnostic procedure or an emergency that requires a stay in the ICU. It applies to everything that goes on from the time a person senses that something is amiss and seeks care from your system, to the point at which your system has provided the best possible care in response. It is relevant to what happens to a patient during a single episode of care, and to how a patient manages a long term, chronic illness across multiple interactions in multiple places.

To establish what is "acceptable" performance, you can measure what you do now to determine the routine variations that occur, and set parameters based on experiences so that most of the predicted variation occurs within these boundaries. These are your tolerances. Even better is to base the parameters on the best performance levels you can find in healthcare, then continue to drive your performance to fall within those limits. Whichever approach you use, the variation that occurs within the boundaries is "noise," the routine ups and downs of normal operations as you've defined them. When something falls outside the tolerances, however, it is a signal, and represents a learning and improvement opportunity.

A signal like this can occur for several reasons. Most often it is a mistake, a measurement error that produces a false signal. This happens frequently in healthcare because the performance measurement systems are rudimentary compared to many other industries. But a signal is not always wrong. It may occur because a team or an individual doesn't know what to do and needs more training. The boundaries may be wrong and need to be adjusted. Perhaps the process needs to be redesigned to be more stable and consistent, especially if "defects" occur more frequently than predicted. Finally, someone or some team may be unwilling or unable to do things as planned. The remedy may be to adjust the process or, more extreme, to replace those who cannot accept the agreed-to processes.

How, then, do you lead the organization in the development of this learning environment? What should you do to make it happen? Below I've described several steps that can help you.

Measure Your Care and the Processes That Deliver It

This is where you start. Without measurement you are guessing. Start small and build to comprehensive metrics for the entire system. Start where there are champions who want to measure what they do to get better. Ideally, measures are readily available; they don't have to be designed or produced on a one-off basis with lots of extra work. But even if special work is required, so be it; you need the data to get better.

Performance measurement should become a central product of the data produced by your IT systems. But because needs change over time, you need the flexibility in those systems that allows you to gather different data at different times to support different objectives.

Identify Best Care Anywhere You Can Find It and Educate Your Organization about How It Works

To know where you stand, you have to find the best level of performance anywhere you can for any particular clinical problem. This must be measurable, not based on reputation or "buzz." And you have to understand how the performance is achieved in order to incorporate it into your system. You also have to establish the criteria for how to get the information needed to verify that it is indeed the "best" performance, as well as to determine what elements can be adapted for use in your setting. A person or group can help find these best performances, but everyone has a role to play as a discovery agent on behalf of the organization.

Don't confuse the "best care possible" and a "best practice." The best performance is the best care you can find anywhere for a particular condition, injury or service. It is real and measurable. "Best Practice," in contrast, usually refers to a standard defined by outside experts, a consensus that may or may not represent the best a particular institution has achieved. You want the best possible, not a consensus, to be your standard.

Use Evidence-Based Analysis to Establish the Boundaries

The simplest form of "evidence" is the collective wisdom of clinicians and staff. By sharing their expertise, the group arrives at a consensus as a starting point for "evidence" based care. This is an improvement over allowing each clinician to do it her way, or of each care episode varying with the combination of clinicians and support staff on duty on a given day. But let's not kid ourselves. This is not good enough. Group consensus is anecdote and bias-based care that may or may not be the best available. Your patients deserve more.

To use evidence this way requires an understanding of its limits and how to deal with those shortcomings. Rarely is there one way of doing things that fits all patient situations. The most we can hope for is good enough evidence for us to establish boundaries for what is likely to work. The evidence allows us to distinguish between acceptable (e.g. evidence based) practices and those that are inconsistent with the available evidence, whatever its quality. Within the boundaries of what is acceptable care defined this way, clinicians use their judgments to tailor care to the individual needs and expectations of each patient. And learning by investigating the signals permits you to modify the boundaries as your evidence accumulates. When clinicians operate outside the boundaries, their leaders can assess whether or not the evidence is correct and boundaries have been established correctly, or additional education is required to move them within the boundaries the group has established.

It is not easy to do good analysis of the evidence. You have to decide when enough is enough in reviewing the data; and you have to do the proper analysis to establish the weight of evidence from different sources. You also need a method to stay abreast of the ever-changing performance bars across healthcare; a cadre of skilled analysts, for example, can support the clinicians in finding and assessing the evidence used to establish or reevaluate the boundaries on an ongoing basis.

To speed the process, you may be inclined to import guidelines produced by others instead of developing your own. Avoid doing so if you can, as these constraints are not likely to engender the commitment you need from the physicians or the workforce as a whole. If your clinicians do this work instead, even something as simple as reviewing and modifying the guidelines developed by others, the limits are self-imposed.

Develop Your Language to Support Learning

What you say about learning carries enormous weight. If you believe it is a key part of a successful transformation, you have to make it the focus of what you talk about in virtually every situation you are in. If things go well, you can point out how learning contributed; if they don't, you can underscore the importance of learning from the mistakes. Of course this doesn't mean that you do not demand superior performance. Someone who makes the same mistake over and over may not have been given the right learning opportunity, may not be able to do the work, or may simply be the wrong person for the job. You have to select the right intervention for the situation.

There are many opportunities to reinforce positive examples. For example, you can support people who have found a best performance outside your organization and successfully introduced it into your organization in spite of the initial resistance they may have encountered. People often earn new certificates or degrees outside normal working hours in order to broaden their perspectives or improve their employability. Acknowledge them. If you look, you see opportunities everywhere. Each time you recognize someone who has learned and improved, you reinforce its importance. When you neglect to do so, on the other hand, you send a subtle message that it isn't as important as your rhetoric suggests.

Establish Rewards and Incentives to Support Learning

In chapter nineteen I discuss how to leverage accountability and incentives to promote your quality agenda. When it comes to learning, you can do this in a number of ways. Save your most powerful rewards for groups that have worked together to do something different or to improve care for patients. It is an opportunity to celebrate the learning and reinforce that most patient care involves groups and teams rather than an individual or two. Groups respond best to immediate, face-to-face acknowledgement. Tell them directly. You don't have to yell and clap, or get on the public address system. The immediacy and intimacy of direct acknowledgement is plenty powerful. A personal letter of thanks can mean a lot too. Formal recognition events can reinforce the importance of both team and individual learning. You can acknowledge the people who have earned degrees while working at the organization. The point is there are myriad ways to reward people for learning, especially when it results in better care.

Establish "Report Backs"

Another tool is to have each person who attends a conference or course outside the organization report back to peers, and where appropriate, to the leadership team and the board of directors. The report should focus on what was learned and what the implications might be for your organization. Like everything else, you have to plan and execute this well to accomplish what you want from it.

In particular the report backs should summarize the context: who sponsored the conference or course? Who spoke or taught? What was the format? What was your assessment of the utility of the meeting or course? Then attention shifts to three core questions: (1) what were the three to five key takeaways from the meeting or course, (2) what were the most important lessons that you learned, and (3) what lessons apply to your organization and how? The discussion that follows should focus on the lessons and their application to your organization. Doing this reinforces the value of learning from sources outside the organization. It gives exposure and accountability to those who use organizational funds and time away to pursue new information. And it plants seeds in the organization with a steady stream of new ideas and different points of view that make it difficult for people to ignore and become increasingly insular over time.

The approach is especially useful for senior team members and for the expanded leadership group. But don't stop there. It is applicable throughout the entire organization. Make sure the reports are first hand, in person, and verbal instead of written. Materials collected at the conferences and courses should be distributed to those who are interested. The summaries of the meetings, the key findings, and the implications should be provided in a discussion, with opportunities to ask questions, seek clarification, and challenge assertions. Above all, you want these report backs to be interactive, engaging the reporter and the audience in an exchange of ideas and discussion of possible applications inside your organization.

Build Collaborative Learning Plans

We learn best what we teach others. To teach well we have to know what is important and explain it in a clear manner that others understand. This is challenging, especially for those without teaching experience. Instead of bringing outsiders into the organization to train your people, develop the skills of insiders to do it yourself. Limit outside instructors to discussions designed to make your people aware of what is happening beyond the walls of your organization, or to make the first introductions of the methods you plan to use. As quickly as possible, though, use your in-house capacity, not only because it's cheaper (it usually is), but because the people who teach are likely to get better at their jobs, and the people who learn are more likely to listen to someone they know.

Establish formal curricula and clear expectations for what is taught and how. Precision is important in both. You'll focus on care integration: the methods used, the findings, the improvements, the results, and the ongoing efforts to make further improvements. You also want a straightforward way to teach these materials, and to evaluate the teaching so that the quality of the teaching starts high and gets better with time. Finally, the learning should emphasize group interactions and participation. The didactic portions of the curriculum should complement the sharing, not the other way around. Done well, the collaborative learning plans should accelerate the changes you seek, as colleagues share their successes and challenges and become increasingly engaged in the improvements.

Once you have established the collaborative inside your organization, you may choose to replicate it for outsiders. Beyond reputation building and helping others, this provides another opportunity for people in your organization to hone their skills and deepen their understanding by teaching. It consumes resources, however, and you have to decide whether or not the returns are worth the investment.

Develop and Maintain the Expertise of the Senior Team, Expanded Leadership Group, and Board of Directors

If you ask your organization to embrace a model of change and methods for making them, all leaders in the organization should be trained to lead these efforts. Once trained, they can teach in the internal training programs and collaborative learning plans. Their commitment of time is evidence of the importance you and your colleagues place on this fundamental building block. To do this you have to invest appropriate resources, and ensure that you and your colleagues are visible as both teachers and students in the ongoing learning processes.

Establish Education Programs for All Staff—Including Physicians—Which Cover Model, Methods, Values, and Expectations

You cannot expect people to function in a new way unless they understand what is expected of them and how they can go about the work to accomplish these objectives. They have to learn and internalize the values of the organization, and the model and methods that define your change process. Most of us share many of the same values, but they may or may not be the ones you expect everyone to internalize in your organization. The starting place for newly hired employees is thorough grounding in these values and expectations, and the consequences for deviating from them. All employees and physicians must learn how to use the methods you have chosen. You have to provide training and support to help people continue to learn as they apply the methods. They learn further by sharing through the collaborative learning plans mentioned above.

As always, this level of education and support requires adequate resources. The training programs must be properly staffed and supported, you may need to backfill for people when they are in their training programs, and you also have to hire the support people for the organization with a proper development and career pathway so they are committed to this work.

Finally, Establish Learning Metrics for Your Performance Dashboard

Your performance dashboard should include measures of how well your learning system works. There is no blueprint for this. You may want to begin with process measures that track how many people have been trained and retrained, how many collaborative learning plans have been established, how many report-backs occur, and the like. As soon as you can, however, you will want your metrics to focus on how rapidly new ideas and improvements make their way into daily operations. You will also want to track how people judge the learning environment by using surveys that assess learning opportunities, support for values related to learning, and the extent to which leaders embody and reinforce the importance of learning in the eyes of the people of the organization, etc. The fact that you ask these same question again and again in the surveys reinforces the importance you place on continuous learning, especially if you link the surveys to visible improvements in your learning systems.

CHAPTER FIFTEEN

TRANSPARENCY

Michael Leonard, MD, as mentioned earlier, played a key role in leading KP's Patient Safety program. He also taught many of us about the value of transparency. During a surgical operation in Denver, CO, in which Mike was the anesthesiologist, he gave his elderly patient the wrong medication as the patient's surgery was nearing completion. Instead of an injection to reverse the effects of the anesthesia and speed the patient's return to consciousness, Mike administered a medication that paralyzed the patient so that, among other things, he was unable to breathe on his own. The medications on Mike's anesthesia tray looked the same: same size and shape, same color labels, and same colored liquid. Fortunately Mike quickly realized what had happened and administered an antidote, and helped the patient breathe until he could do it on his own. After a long delay, the gentleman was sent to post-op recovery fully recovered from this near miss.

As soon as the patient was settled, Mike sought out the family to tell them what had happened. After reassuring them that their family member was doing fine, he described the near-fatal error, why it had happened, and what he had done to reverse the effects. He had trouble holding back his tears. The family responded by thanking him for his honesty, expressing their gratitude for the care he had provided, and comforting him until he regained his composure. Mike promoted the policy of immediate communication with patients and families when errors and near misses occur, transparency that KP tries to emulate every day.

Transparency is a centerpiece of the patient-centered organization, contributes to the culture of engagement and learning you seek to build, and is an important building block for creating trust and confidence within the communities you serve. This is a "no secrets" approach. It means you let people see what you do and how you perform, what you do well and what you don't, without censure or limits. It is all out there, good, bad, or indifferent.

How much transparency is necessary? You have to answer the question for your organization. You have to start by deciding whether or not truth and openness matter in healthcare; whether you are better off when you tell the truth or if you hedge or only talk about the good things? It's a legitimate question. Our advisors urge caution. The specter of trial lawyers looms large. None of us wants to put our organization in jeopardy. The wiser approach might seem to selectively share information, to screen and censure what could be damaging.

I believe you are better off being open. If you are consistent, and if you are careful to place the information in the proper context for your audience, most people respond as you would hope. In healthcare especially, people appreciate the consistency with which you provide information, your willingness to share the good and bad news, and your commitment to improving performance every day. The real challenge is to show those improvements. You can't stand still and expect the public or your employees, and least of all patients, to remain committed to the future of the organization just because you've been open with them. You also have to be smart. You must decide when to release information and, especially if the news is not good, how to lay the groundwork to ready key audiences and make sure the people who receive the news are well enough informed to interpret it accurately.

Transparency like this creates an important competitive standard. Once you reveal your performance, every health system you compete against must follow, or admit that they don't have the information or won't share it if they do. Once you show good and bad results and what you are doing to improve, others will have a harder time getting away with publishing just their good results. They will be held to the same standard, not right away, but over time.

This happened at Norton Health System in Louisville, KY, which since the late 1980s has made their quality indicator results public. Today their quality metrics are available online for anyone to see. Have they suffered as a result? Not according to Steve Williams, the CEO. He reports that there has been a decline in malpractice actions against the organization and increased scrutiny of the other systems in their community. The organization has a reputation for honesty and has improved steadily. The result? Demand for care and market share has increased.

As you consider how to implement your no secrets policies, it is helpful to consider how it will apply to three different audiences: patients, the people of the organization, and the communities you serve.

Transparency with Patients

Your intent is to establish objectives for what patients should expect, what they should receive in their interactions with the system, and what your performance is in practice compared to those objectives.

The patient covenant or promise. Many organizations display a covenant, a promise to the patient, often called a Patient Bill of Rights, in waiting rooms and public spaces. Most of these address issues of dignity, privacy, and confidentiality. Some describe the information the patients should expect. Few, however, talk about transparency. You are well served to do so, to promise that there will be no secrets about their care, or the care processes they experience, or the performance of the organization and the clinicians who practice in it. It is a promise to share what they can expect and what happens in the care they receive, good or bad; and that there will be no surprises. In the event there are problems, including mistakes, you commit to providing immediate explanations so the patient is not left confused or fearful. If a mistake is made, they will know about it. In sum, you promise that you will do everything you can to help them understand what they will experience and to be clear about what actually happens. You also promise that they will understand what they are charged and why.

Performance expectations. You want to be sure every patient knows what to expect from your physicians, nurses, clinicians, support people, and the organization itself in terms of her care experience.

- **About care:** A common complaint of patients is that they don't know what to expect, they can't get straight answers to their questions, and they are unsure what is happening from one moment to the next. You want to ensure that she receives the information she needs to understand what is happening at every step of the way and why. She will not be surprised. If something unexpected does occur, she learns why as quickly as possible. She should have all the information she needs to make intelligent choices about her care, and will have the final say in what is done.

  To inform patients this way requires careful attention to the values that underlie this commitment, and to the methods used to talk with patients about their care. It is not a simple matter of establishing a form for informed consent or creating the perfect video to explain a particular procedure. Nor is it just making sure everyone who interacts with patients knows this is important. To build the skills to be transparent this way takes education, feedback, evaluation, and improvement in the same continuous cycle that we want to see throughout the care delivery process itself.

- **About performance:** To choose their care wisely, including the physicians and teams that they rely on, patients need to know how well the system and these physicians perform. They have a right to real-time data to be able to make informed decisions about their care. Nothing about performance should be off limits (except for personal problems among clinicians).

- **About preventable errors:** Patients have a right to full disclosure and an apology when a preventable error occurs, whether or not it results in harm or death. Your lawyers will probably tell you not to do this, and your medical staff may resist too. In my experience, honesty and transparency like this actually increases the patient's confidence that you are trying to do the right thing. If your physicians and clinicians and support staff always sit down with a patient and their family when a mistake has been made, apologize for it, and describe what has been done to ensure that it never happens again, patients seldom take legal action. They may want compensation if the accident is sufficiently grave or the damage permanent. If so, it is important to treat a settlement in the same spirit of openness and honesty. Keep these discussions out of the adversarial legal world and in yours for as long as you can by doing the right thing for the patient and family.

Some people are litigious no matter what you do. Most are not, though, and it is a mistake to build an approach on the exception instead of the rule. In my experience, most people know when you are being honest and forthcoming, and they can see the anguish you feel when you fail them. They want to be treated fairly for what they have gone through but don't expect you to be their winning lottery ticket. With time and experience, you develop a feel for when you are heading toward formal litigation. When this happens, you have to protect your institution, and the rules of transparency may not apply.

Like so many other things, it takes learning, feedback, and support to do this well. It is hard for anyone to admit to a mistake, especially so when the patient has been harmed or lost. If you are like most in healthcare, you have received little, if any, training in how to do this. You know that avoidable errors extract a heavy toll on the providers, as well as the patients. And because these conversations with patients and their families are so often emotional, the commitment to transparency produces an even greater burden. Fortunately a rich literature exists on the subject and should be required reading for you and your leadership team as you create the training programs, and the support and feedback systems you need to implement this expectation.

- **About metrics:** Finally, it is important to establish metrics that help care teams determine whether or not their patients understand what to expect, why things happen as they do, and what the performance expectations are. The teams need to determine where to set the bar initially, and then be held accountable for the continuous improvement in performance over time. Organization-level metrics about these matters are not particularly helpful. It has to be more granular, at the point of care and focused on whether or not the teams are improving their care. If patients can be involved in helping set the expectations and designing the tools to provide the information, and if they can be involved in assessing how well the team is meeting those expectations, so much the better. Your job is to set the process in motion, then through regular interactions and measurement, determine that the teams do what is expected on a day-in and day-out basis.

Transparency for the People of the Organization

The audience for your second level of transparency is your workforce.

Performance. Nothing should be hidden about the performance of the organization and the individuals in it. Everything should be open to scrutiny: results and improvements in quality, safety, service, and financial performance. These should be available month after month, good and bad.

You cannot expect to reach full transparency on day one; you have to grow into it. In some instances you must "blind" the results for individual clinicians. They might each be able to see their own results but know only how they measure up to the other clinicians as a group. You may start with results for teams and departments, letting the individual groups decide how far to go in revealing and reviewing individual results. The goal is to reach a level of transparency that provides everyone in the organization with insight into how well the organization performs, how well their area of activity and focus is doing to meet expectations, and how effectively they have improved their performance over time.

Issues and decisions. In the daily crunch of running an institution, issues and decisions arise at a hectic pace. Some are false alarms or minor, many turn out not to be as critical as they first appeared to be, some are important. It is impossible to inform the organization about every one of them. You have to filter the information, not to color what people hear but to limit it to important matters so people are not distracted from their everyday work. You can use two guidelines for this. First is whether or not people need the information to do their jobs. Clearly, information about performance is central to what they do; they have to know about performance to improve it. The second is whether or not they need to know to plan their futures. They have a right to know what to expect from the institution in terms of financial and performance health so they can make the necessary adjustments in their own lives.

A straightforward, simple, direct approach is preferable when you share information. You want to convey the important facts, let people know the alternatives you considered, and provide the reasons for your actions. People should also know what might happen to them. And always, you want to be sure there is an opportunity for people to ask their questions. Sharing like this is a two-way street.

Transparency is about keeping people in the loop. It is a commitment to building trust, to the idea that most people will accept information when it is provided honestly and without colorations to make it appear better or more positive than it is. It is about being honest about your mistakes so they will be open about theirs. Each time you share you have to pay attention to the context and the consequences. You have to anticipate how people are likely to react and be prepared to address those reactions when they arise. If the news about performance is bad or the financial status of the organization is shaky, people are likely to be concerned about their futures. You have to be prepared to respond. You also have to be honest about what you have chosen to share and how you have shared it. You have to admit when you cannot say more if this is the case. Transparency is a standard for all that happens in the organization. The way you choose to live it sends powerful messages about who you are and what you stand for, and creates the culture that enables those you rely on to be equally transparent with you.

An important element of the original Kaiser Permanente Labor Management Partnership in 1997 was the commitment to open the financial books of the organization. Management agreed to share financial results with the participating Unions on a regular basis. The value of this became clear when labor contracts came up for negotiation. Instead of the unproductive finger pointing of traditional negotiations, the participants focused on the real choices they had because they knew what the fiscal realities of the organization were. The provisions provided labor and management with conditions they could work with, while the duration of the agreement, seven years, meant the partners could turn their attention to the more critical issues of patient care quality and worker safety that required their shared participation.

Transparency with the Public

The third audience for transparency is the public. Openness with the public is an important goal for an institution like yours that plays such a central role in the lives of the communities you serve. It is usually a competitive advantage and it changes the conversations in and out of your organization. If you are transparent about your performance, good and bad, it can force your competitors to do the same. It raises the bar. People come to expect this candor. Your willingness to be transparent signals that you are unafraid of your mistakes because you learn from them. Candor and honesty allow you to figure out what you need to do better. And that commitment, that unrelenting search for better outcomes and better care, is what ultimately sets you apart.

As with patients and the people of the organization, you have to be thoughtful about this. You have to think carefully about what you say and how you say it, about when and where you tell your story. This does not mean dishonesty or half-truth telling. It means that you are consistent and steady, direct, candid about the good and bad, and fierce about making things better. When you make a mistake, you don't hide behind legalese, you don't pretend everything's fine, you don't downplay the seriousness. Importantly, you also don't make excuses. You fix it. Every time. And you communicate that too.

Another part of transparency here is to invite members of the community to join the work the institution does. You want to be sure to cast a wide net. Transparency works best for people outside the institution when they see and touch it, when they see you in action inside as well as outside the organization, demonstrating your commitment to openness and candor, sharing the good and bad in multiple settings with different groups.

With this in mind, there are several specific areas to consider.

Performance. Similar to the focus inside the organization, you want to provide regular, accessible information to the public about your performance. You may want to share those aspects most important to the general public: quality of care, patient safety, and service. You may also want to track the ways your work improves the efficiency of care and lowers the costs. This is a trickier message to craft for the reasons already mentioned. But with believable data and consistent language, you can hammer home the core intent of your strategy: to provide the best care possible, to include patients and their families in the design of that care, and as a result, continuously work to eliminate the waste and unnecessary care that both harms and drives costs so high.

You don't become transparent by issuing a one-time performance report card, or participating in national surveys, or admitting publicly that a mistake has been made and describing what you will do to prevent it from happening again. Transparency is a commitment, a collection of actions over a long period of time. You build a reputation slowly, one step at a time, demonstrating it by what you do and say and how you act over months and years.

Involvement. As noted already, there is no better way for the public to witness your commitment than by working with you. If you are transparent inside the organization and with your patients, the public will see this when they become involved. There are several ways to do this. You can invite members of the community to comment on a particular project in a one-off engagement. This can be helpful in planning and executing the plans for a new building or an expanded hospital. You can ask community representatives to review your expansion plans or your intentions for services over the coming years. Again this can be a one-off arrangement. The more effective interactions, though, occur when members of the community join teams from the organization to analyze and plan strategy, or to develop specific plans for new services or facilities, or to engage in annual goal-setting exercises that the institution conducts. In general, the more engagement you have across a range of activities, the better for opening the doors and sharing what occurs within your institution. Rather than telling them what you do, they can see for themselves, and they watch you and your leadership team in action, walking the walk, as it were, in addition to talking the talk.

You may also want to ask representatives from the community to join committees of the board of directors. Special ad-hoc committees can help with particularly visible issues in the community at large. Kaiser Permanente had a controversial policy in place for many years that required members to use mediation instead of litigating their malpractice claims through the tort system. Trial lawyers disliked this policy, and some consumer advocates criticized it for a perceived organizational bias. Even the state legislature in California became involved from time to time. Our view was different: we saw it as fair, balanced, and more often beneficial to the plaintiff than the tort pathway. Mediation also was a means to avoid the negative publicity and huge settlements that can occur in the few cases that actually go to jury trial.

The board of directors and the leadership team realized, though, that our lack of responsiveness was eroding our credibility. A Blue Ribbon Committee was created to review our approach and suggest revisions as appropriate. It was chaired by a retired federal judge, and included a former California state legislator and the president of a local community foundation. Our commitment to them was fourfold: (1) provide access to all data they needed to carry out their work, (2) freedom for them to make whatever recommendations they believed were appropriate to change our system up to and including abandoning the approach altogether, (3) freedom to communicate their findings and recommendations to the public and the press after they had shared their report with the KP leadership, and (4) implementation of those recommendations the senior leaders and board of directors agreed with, and full disclosure as to why those not implemented were excluded.

The outcome was better than we dared hope. The committee carried out its work in the public eye. They praised our openness in providing the data they needed and reinforced the value of mediation for both individuals and our organization. They were critical of the way we ran the mediation system, however, and made a number of helpful recommendations to strengthen it. All of the recommendations were accepted without change. And when the committee released their report to the public, the organization was able to communicate what we intended to do at the same time.

Candor. You may be familiar with the case in which Johnson & Johnson responded to the threat of tainted Tylenol, a highly profitable product, by removing every bottle from the shelves across the entire country until the problem could be resolved. They did this, they explained, because of their core values about honesty and safety. By admitting that something might be wrong and taking action that carried significant short-term economic consequences, they reinforced their reputation for excellence, honesty, and candor, and their credibility as a company soared.

It's an important object lesson for all of us in healthcare. Our typical response is to hem and haw, stonewall, hedge, and gloss over mistakes or problems. We use "company speak" that is sterile and devoid of emotion: "perhaps," or "it appears that…," or "…we are looking into it…," etc. Sometimes this approach works; the problem fades away and the attention shifts. Sometimes hunkering down, offering vague responses, then riding things out is the right thing to do, but it also risks damaging the public's perception about you. It can look like you are afraid of the truth, and that the public is too ignorant or untrustworthy for you to tell them what is really happening. Rather than building bridges to the community and the people you serve, these words can separate you, creating distance that is hard to bridge.

Usually candor is better: straightforward, unadorned, unambiguous language that conveys exactly what has happened, why, and what you intend to do about it. No frills. No excuses. No ducking responsibility. It helps too if you can get in front of an issue before it becomes public, or before the press begins to investigate what is happening. That way you can convey what you want without having to respond to the questions—even accusations—that are often the starting place for reporters or the public at large.

Transparency, then, is the third tool of the leader in building the new operating capabilities into your organization. Whether working with patients, relating to the people of the organization, or addressing the public and the community, the principle of "no secrets" reinforces your commitment to quality and safety, as well as to learning and improvement.

CHAPTER SIXTEEN

INNOVATION

"...openness and connectivity may, in the end, be more

valuable to innovation than purely competitive mechanisms."

– Steven Johnson, *Where Good Ideas Come From*, 2010

A few years ago Asian manufacturers, especially in China, began to produce low cost, lower functionality electronic measurement instruments for the emerging markets throughout the world. They gained traction quickly, and leaders at Agilent Technologies believed they posed a real threat to Agilent's long-term leadership in the field. The company had a history of failed efforts to build simpler, less costly instruments. Engineers preferred to focus on building better instruments with new capabilities. When asked to create cheaper products, they crammed high-end functionality into less expensive boxes. Often the company had ceded the lower end markets to the new entrants. There was also a concern that low-end products would cannibalize their profitable existing ones, so management, marketing, and sales leaders were usually negative about these efforts.

Bill Sullivan, the CEO of Agilent, and his team were unwilling to repeat this pattern. They believed they had the engineering, manufacturing, and marketing capabilities to design and sell low-cost instruments that could win against these new competitors. They also believed that doing so would expand their market instead of cannibalize existing product lines; and they argued that the low-end instruments would familiarize manufacturers with Agilent so they would be more likely to purchase high-end products as their companies grew. A gifted engineer and manager, Gooi Soon Chai, was assigned to head up this effort in Penang, Malaysia, where he had already assembled a team of top flight managers, engineers, and manufacturing experts to run the Agilent operations there. With earmarked funding and a dedicated team located far from Agilent's traditional engineering strength in the US, Gooi and his team designed new lines of low cost instruments for the rapidly emerging markets. He was challenged with difficult targets for product introductions, market growth, and profitability. Sullivan and Gooi's immediate boss, Ron Nersesian, met regularly with him and his team to track progress. And unlike previous attempts, this one was successful.

Within two years the Penang team had prototyped, and begun to manufacture and sell new lines of low-cost, lower-functionality test and measurement products that were well received in the target markets. Many were portable and easy to use. Functional requirements were defined by the customers and designed accordingly. Production costs were low and prices were highly competitive as a result. Further, all the design, prototyping, manufacturing, and marketing was done in Penang by local engineers and managers. Agilent leaders had successfully disrupted the company's traditional approach to product design and manufacturing, and tapped a new source of creativity for the company in a rapidly growing part of the world. They were able to serve new markets, and they created a brand that promised further migration into high-end Agilent products as the markets expanded along with the economies of SE Asia and the BRICS countries.

The never-ending care improvement cycle—your focus on operational excellence—is how you deliver the best care possible day after day, year after year. To ensure that you do not fall behind disruptive shifts in care delivery, however, you also must bring new capabilities and non-traditional solutions into your system. Improvement isn't enough, in other words, especially not in today's environment. You need more. Traditional care systems must improve their performance to remain competitive, and they must be prepared to respond to innovative solutions others may introduce that have the potential to create a completely different race.

Consider, for example, what happens when a delivery system creates a back or spine care system designed to treat patients more effectively and return them to work more quickly at substantially lower cost than the traditional models can. Instead of six weeks to return to work, most patients return to full function in two weeks at two-thirds the cost of the traditional model. Employers flock to this new solution. This is more than an incremental change, a simple improvement. It is disruptive because it is so attractive that employers will chose to contract exclusively with it at the expense of those who offer the traditional care.

Or think about how valuable it would be to screen for pre-clinical disease using accurate diagnostic tools delivered directly to consumers in shopping centers, homes, or at the worksite. Imagine that these screening tools could allow the consumer to discover the presence of early stage illness before symptoms or traditional signs of the illness make their appearance for the clinician to see. Imagine as well that the test results would be available in a matter of minutes, performed by a lab technician on a portable machine at a cost of less than one hundred dollars per screen. This, too, is a disruptive innovation that would change the game; a new diagnostic paradigm that would shift care away from physician's offices, clinics, and hospitals, and provide consumers with a different way to get answers to their questions. It would also be cheap enough that individuals could pay for it out of pocket. And it would reduce demand for traditional physician and hospital services. It would also shift "control" over how consumers access the formal care system. Instead of going through their physician, consumers and potential patients could go directly from screening to referral specialists as needed. The screening system would do the triage instead of a physician or an emergency room.

Both examples are real. The first is described by Maureen Bisognano and Charles Kenney in *Pursuing the Triple Aim*. It is the endpoint of a two-stage innovation led by Intel and Virginia Mason physicians in the Seattle, WA, area and modified further in Washington County, Oregon, in collaboration with local physician leaders. The new front-end, disease screening system is under development as this book is being written, led by a biotechnology company and a major public company in partnership with a delivery system that shares an interest in building a population-based screening and triage system in front of their traditional medical care solutions. It remains to be seen whether or not this will work, but even if it fails, someone else will figure out how to put these pieces together so it does.

And that is the point. Advances in medical science and technologies, coupled with those in communications and information technology, are the substrate for innovation in healthcare. Fueled by limitations in our ability to meet current and projected demands for care, entrepreneurs and willing investors are looking for alternatives. These innovations are happening now all around you. As a leader, you need both performance improvement and innovation to transform your organization; Performance improvement is not enough. Nor can you assume that innovations alone will secure your future, that you don't have to invest in improved performance because innovations will pave the way for you. Most innovations fall short of their promise, after all, and take a long time to deliver when they are successful. It is possible to do both, but of all the challenges you face, managing successful improvement and innovation efforts is among the most difficult.

Improvement, as I've emphasized again and again, is hard work. The relentless assessment of how well you are doing now, the never-ending search for better ways to do your work, the endless cycle of discovery, testing, measurement, and improvement, is rewarding and exhausting. To do this across an organization consistently enough to deliver superior care requires an unrelenting drive to overcome the forces that protect the status quo. Now think about introducing innovations that can disrupt these carefully designed solutions. That's challenging! But to secure your future, you have to do both.

Innovation begins with a state of mind, just like transparency and learning, a willingness to learn, try new things, and take appropriate risks while acting with discipline and restraint to ensure that the innovations produce the desired results. It requires strength of purpose to deal with the barriers that impede the implementation of these new solutions. And it requires a commitment to the idea that your future depends on both innovations and improvement to deliver the best care possible. You must find the language that convinces your partners to join you. That's where you start. Then you must decide how to address several general issues.

General Considerations

What Kind of Innovation? Clinicians, support staff, and patients need to work collaboratively to deliver consistently excellent care through their continuous improvement efforts. A subset of them is likely to be motivated to try more radical solutions, something that changes care in more profound ways. They need support and funding to carry out this work because it lies outside the day-to-day improvement environment. If the innovation proves effective, you will want to work with the innovators and thought leaders to move it into the ongoing operation. Added to these one-off opportunities are directed innovations designed to disrupt old ways of working: new treatments, new care delivery processes, new business models, etc. These are planned, purposeful initiatives that complement the improvement efforts and spontaneous innovations.

In-house innovations are likely to be the most immediately relevant to your organization, but you have to make sure they are appropriately led, staffed, and financed if they are to have the impact you seek. If you lack the resources for doing this, you can opt to find innovations outside your system. You can even go one step further and invest in venture or private equity firms that focus on care organization and delivery.

They can provide a window into a broad array of innovations, some of which you may choose to test in your organization. But they are a controversial way to innovate: you pay steep prices to get in, you have to review a host of opportunities to find the very few that could be relevant to your organization, and your financial returns, especially from a venture investment, are likely to be volatile at best.

You have a choice of directed or spontaneous innovation. In a directed innovation program like the one described at Agilent, you would establish specific innovation targets for the program. Then you would establish your priorities, your budgets, and your staffing accordingly, and hold the programs accountable for accomplishing what they've agreed to do. If you select the path of spontaneous innovation, you must build a capacity to look for promising ideas inside and outside the organization, and to connect people so that they can exchange their ideas. In truth you need both. There is an important role for planned innovation activities that focus on specific priorities, while innovations that occur more spontaneously are often more interesting and helpful. You also need to find innovations outside your organization, either to incorporate or adapt them, or to develop defenses if they threaten your markets and your future.

Steven Johnson observes that the number of useful ideas and innovations increases as the number of connections increases among people. He concludes that an essential component of an innovation program is the infrastructure that enables such connections: an information system that helps people share and discuss ideas, build on one another's thinking, and eventually, plan innovations that can be reviewed by the leadership or the formal Innovation Program for funding and support. In addition you must build a culture that invests in and supports innovations, especially those that disrupt the status quo, however painful that may be; and an organizational framework that guides, reviews and helps disseminate the innovation effort.

Guiding Principles

A successful innovation system is guided by several principles:

Protection. The system must be protected from the forces in the organization that squash new ideas before they can take hold. You do this with separate funding, independent staffing, distinct oversight, and in some cases, a direct reporting relationship to the CEO and the board of directors.

Accountability. The system must be held accountable for delivering results that matter. This can't be a playpen for some lucky souls, or a pasture for the poor performers or soon-to-retires. It is too important. The results must be measured, the funding sufficient to carry out the work, and the results reviewed by the leaders to determine whether or not to incorporate the innovation into the mainstream of the organization.

Support. The innovation efforts need your unwavering support, and that of your leadership team, and the board of directors. There will be push back, even conflict, especially as innovations move from development to implementation. Traditional relationships may be affected, power won and lost, and established patterns of control shattered. You will have a lot of explaining and listening to do to ensure that you don't lose the benefits of the innovations, or that the organization doesn't stumble as it tries to integrate the innovations into routine practice.

Outside Expertise. Outsiders selected for their experience and insights expand the net you cast to find promising innovations elsewhere in healthcare and bring different perspectives to your in-house innovation efforts. They must be selected with care to ensure that the time you invest to educate them is worth the effort. You, in turn, want their time to be well used, and to give them something in return: perhaps a financial stake, non-financial rewards, or whatever can strengthen their relationship with your organization.

Language. As with so many aspects of leadership, your innovation effort requires clear language about what it is, why it is important, what is expected of it, how it will affect the larger organization, and how you expect people of the organization to engage with it. The rationale must be grounded in the emerging world as you see it, the same world, by the way, that requires the performance improvements you have highlighted.

Organization

Apart from the general principles just described, how do you organize a successful innovation effort? Like most of the suggestions in this book, it has to fit your circumstances. There is no "right" answer. There are elements, however, that should be considered, whatever approach you take.

Visibility. Your effort should be viewed as a core element of your organization. It needs to be visible in its own right and as an integral part of the organization. It doesn't matter if it is an office, a department, or an institute. People need to know it exists and what you expect it to deliver. Creating the expectation that everyone will be engaged in innovative behavior, or that individuals and teams will develop innovations in addition to their focus on improvement, is insufficient. The press of daily work will overwhelm most innovative thinking before it can get off the ground. You need to appoint a visible leader for the effort, provide a clear charge that reflects the strategy of the organization, create expectations for what the leader and the innovation effort will deliver, and establish a disciplined review of progress to share throughout the organization. Similar to the leaders of the quality improvement efforts, the innovation leader should make regular reports to the board of directors.

Leadership. The effort requires a credible leader who reports directly to you or another member of your leadership team. That leader must be able to work with the managers and clinicians throughout the organization to ensure that the spontaneous opportunities are captured and the implementation of new ideas can occur. In other words, this effort must be viewed as part of the daily work of the organization. The leader you choose has to be someone who can make that goal a reality.

Funding. The innovation effort is a strategic investment and should be funded appropriately. It cannot be an afterthought, something done on the cheap, a "nice but not necessary" part of the annual budget. It is preferable to allocate a proportion of your annual budget to the program, a percentage of the total budget, for example, 5 percent or 10 percent in a given year; or an absolute dollar level that you are willing to support. You want to be sure to commit to a three to five year program rather than funding it year to year. This ensures that the efforts have sufficient time to develop without the immediate threat of defunding hanging over them. You also need to budget for implementation. A common mistake is to under-invest: too little financial support, leadership support, and time, in effect setting these new solutions up to fail before they can deliver on their promise.

You want to encourage the program leaders to find outside sources of funds to supplement those you provide if possible. This can be tricky, however. You don't want to lose control of the innovations by, in effect, selling them to others. Nor do you want to enrich the individuals at the expense of the organization. You need clear rules of the road for outside investments if you decide to encourage their use. Fortunately many academic medical centers and research laboratories have addressed this concern and can provide some guidance. If you are a not-for-profit organization, you must be mindful of the limits on revenues from profit-making enterprises. These vary by state, in addition to the customary limits established by the IRS.

The innovation system helps you shape your organization over time. Like your improvement efforts, your innovations are designed to find new ways to deliver the best care possible, strengthen your competitive position, and develop the capabilities you need to respond to different futures. Unlike the improvements, though, the innovations are directed to the disruptive forces in healthcare, the forces that require you to abandon traditional ways of delivering care, traditional business models, and even your traditional networks and collaborators. To build the capacity to innovate into your organization, you must provide the leadership that helps your people embrace innovation, organize the effort appropriately, and support and fund it at a level sufficient to be an integral part of your strategy.

You also have to provide sufficient resources for implementing the innovations you decide to extend throughout the organization. This is the hardest part of innovation. To be successful you have to displace the traditional care models and delivery solutions, and in so doing, disrupt long-standing patterns of status, relationships, and work among the very partners you rely on to do the hard work of improving the care they provide today. It can be done, but you have to approach the effort with great care, careful organization, repeated explanations, and steady leadership and financial support to help the people in the organization make this difficult transformation.

CHAPTER SEVENTEEN

INFORMATION

Rolling out an information system is seldom easy. The system-wide electronic medical record (EMR) at KP is a case in point. A decision about which EMR to choose was made four times in the course of the initial eight years of the rollout effort. The first was to ask the leaders of the region's individual EMR efforts to choose the best of each for a total KP solution. After two years no progress had been made. In 1996 the Program leaders selected the IBM system in the Colorado region as the most suitable choice for the entire Program. A year later the Southern California Permanente Medical Group raised enough questions to force a reexamination of the entire decision process. The Colorado-IBM solution was reaffirmed, and the rollout continued. Two years later the Northwest region objected so strongly to the decision to replace their successful EPIC system that the IT Steering Committee felt compelled to review their original decision once more. Again the Colorado solution emerged as the system of choice. In 2002 when George Halvorson became CEO, he asked the IT leadership team and Steering Committee to examine the status of the off-the-shelf EMR solutions. Based on that review, the Colorado solution was replaced with the upgraded and strengthened EPIC solution. Between 2002 and 2012 the EPIC was rolled out through all the regions; from start to finish the process lasted sixteen years.

It took time to help each physician learn to incorporate computer terminals and a computerized record system into the daily flow of a busy practice. This new choreography couldn't be rushed. Multiple changes had to be made in the system to accommodate the requirements of different specialists. A rollout like this is unprecedented in its scope. Not only does it connect eighteen thousand Permanente physicians, it also provides online access for every member to their medical information, the pharmacy refill system, and by e-mail to their physicians. The expense has been huge, an estimated $6 billion to bring the system to its current state. But the benefits are enormous for patients and members, for physicians and clinicians, and for researchers who have an unprecedented and growing clinical database that can be connected to the Program's large genetic data bank as well as other research programs.

It is a sobering reminder of how hard it is to make and implement a decision in any system where competing interests have so much influence. It certainly was tempting to cut our losses and give in to the resistance. Concerns arose continuously about the costs, forcing us to review budgets again and again to be sure our approach was the best possible. Push back about the choice of the Colorado solution was not unexpected. We relied on a transparent, credible, and objective process to convince the participants that the choice made sense, and each time the decision was reviewed, the decision stood up. When the new capacities of the off-the-shelf solutions were validated, the Program leaders pivoted to a better solution. Key to the successful rollout was the Permanente Federation, which had built a strong staff to help physicians and adapt decision-support capabilities developed by the Care Management Institute to the new EMR.

A twenty-first century healthcare delivery system cannot function without timely, useful information. Today's information technologies are the pipes and reservoirs that store and move this information from one place to another, anytime and anywhere it is needed. And they provide the analytic heft to turn the mountains of data into usable form. It would be easiest to start with a blank slate, but few have that luxury. If yours is like most healthcare organizations, you have many legacy systems that have grown, like Topsy, over time. They may not talk to one another, but they contain important data and represent sunk costs and ongoing operational expenses that cannot be ignored. The "Meaningful Use" requirements to receive stimulus funding and avoid Medicare-related penalties are additional considerations. How you deal with your legacy systems, the regulatory requirements, and your imperative to build your new delivery capabilities is an art form. Much is dependent on your legacy systems and how far along you are in complying with the various requirements. You have to tailor your solutions to the needs and capabilities of your organization.

It helps to have an overarching framework to make sense of the issues, a view of what information is needed, for what purposes, where, and when, as well as an idea of how your information needs will evolve over the coming decade. Otherwise you are like the ship captain navigating through thick fog without instruments. The information you require must satisfy several objectives, and the sequence in which you build them should depend on your circumstances and your capital and operational constraints.

Patients

An important capability in your new delivery system is to give patients access to the information they need to stay as healthy as possible and to manage their illnesses well. They also need the right information in order to use their time and that of the healthcare professionals appropriately, to answer questions about their care, to arrange for their care and medications, and to track their progress over time. To accomplish these goals, several elements are required:

- Access to information about the medications they are taking, the clinical problems they are dealing with, the key diagnostic findings (historical data, physical data, lab and imaging data, etc.), reports of key consultations, etc.

- Anytime, anywhere access to information and advice that helps them answer their questions about their health, including deciding whether to do something, or not, how, and where to access the care system when it is necessary.

- Online messaging with personal physicians and other clinicians, pharmacy reordering, appointment scheduling, referral management, etc.

- Online contact from the health system to individual members and patients as needed.

Clinicians

You may have already invested in information systems, including EMRs, to help the physicians, and possibly other clinicians, conduct their clinical practices. This is a good start, but it is far from sufficient to meet the information challenges you have. In the context of the care transformation, the information that clinicians need is specific and critically important.

- Every clinician needs access to historic, laboratory, imaging, and other diagnostic and therapeutic data to diagnose, treat, and follow her patients.

- All treating clinicians need access to the same information as well as to the work each is doing on behalf of the patient. This includes: work up information (history, physical, lab, imaging, etc.), preliminary and final diagnostic and treatment plans, and agreements reached by the team, with the patient and family as appropriate, about the future plans (therapies, follow up, behavior changes, etc.).
- Registries of patients with different conditions/illnesses for whom tracking and adjusting care is essential to achieve the best outcomes; and collective data is useful for managing each subpopulation.

- Online order entry: lab, imaging, referrals, support services, in-patient orders, etc.

- Evidence-based clinical decision criteria and support materials, as well as background technical reference resources.

- Communications systems that link clinicians to one another and to their patients, enabling real-time consultations and discussions about diagnostic findings and interpretations, treatment alternatives, and preferred clinical care plans.

Support Personnel

Support personnel and their departments also have specific information needs to be able to provide their services in a timely and efficient way:

- Access to orders and appropriate information from clinicians.

- Two-way communication between support staff and providers, as well as among support staff themselves.

- Scheduling and patient tracking system to maximize efficiency and maintain visibility into where patients are at all times while in the care system.

Performance

Leaders, managers, and clinicians need real-time information about the performance of the system at all levels: what it is doing at any given time; who is doing it; how much time it is taking to do it; how actual performance compares to target performance; how observed compares with projected performance for improvement projects, and so forth. Specific information includes:

- **Volume and Use:** How many patients? What characteristics? What problems or conditions? What treatments? What lengths of stay? What condition returns to ER within thirty days? Etc.

- **Quality/Safety:** actual care provided, outcomes achieved compared to targets, best-performance levels, success in meeting improvement targets, etc.

- **Service:** responses of patients and families to the interactions they have with the care system and the care they receive. Success in meeting improvement targets, etc.

- **Costs:** unit costs, production costs, total costs v. revenues. Success in meeting improvement targets.

The key to performance data is transparency, the widespread availability of performance information in a no-secrets way.

Improvement and Learning

When care is simple, the information requirements to support improvement and learning are too. But they increase rapidly as care becomes more complex and as more caregivers and locations are involved. The challenge of linking these components is substantial. To aggregate information from these sources into coherent pictures of what is happening is more challenging still. And most difficult is to develop the analytic capabilities that enable you and your organization to use the information to examine and modify clinical insights and practices, manage the populations you serve, and ensure that your organization is healthy and growing.

Revenues

To be paid, regardless of who is paying, the system has to generate information about the services it provides and who it provides them to.

Payers range all over the map in their criteria for what they cover, how much they pay, for example, so the system needs access to these plans to determine what to bill for. To justify what your system charges, you need valid service data from throughout the system and from the large number of encounters and actions that occur during any particular episode of care. The requirements are less onerous in a contract or bundled payment system, and even less so in a full capitation payment model. The granular, cost-based justifications for charges in the fee-for-service (FFS) world are not necessary in the other payment models, at least not to justify payment. They are, however, important in tracking the work and production effectiveness of your system.

Regulatory and Legal Compliance

Every system needs information to meet regulatory and legal requirements and challenges. Like other enterprises, healthcare systems cannot defend what they do by asking the courts, the regulators, and the patients to "trust them." It doesn't work that way. For the most part, the regulatory requirements can be met with the information you collect to run and improve your system. Similarly, your ability to defend yourself against legal action often depends on your ability to document performance and demonstrate continuous improvement.

As you think about your road map, you want to design your solutions so that you: (1) collect the information once and reuse it for multiple purposes; (2) move it seamlessly and quickly from one provider to another, and from one place to another; (3) store it securely and efficiently, expand it as necessary, and access and use it easily and efficiently; (4) aggregate and analyze it in increasingly complex ways as the data grows and information requirements expand.

These categories and data characteristics can serve as a road map for the information you need to lead your organization through this delivery system transformation. Having a full picture is essential for building the systems and supporting technologies you will require. No one information system does all of these things; as a result, you are likely to end up with a patchwork quilt of solutions to meet your needs.

As you do, remember a few basic rules.

- **Keep it simple.** If you don't understand it, it is unlikely the people in the organization will either.

- **Fix your processes.** If you haven't organized your care processes properly, you will spend far more resources than necessary to obtain data that provides little insight into where improvements are needed. We all know the adage, "Garbage in, garbage out."

- **Forget what others are doing.** Don't be a lemming. You have to decide what's best for your organization at the stage you are and with the legacy systems you already have. You should learn all you can from others, but in the final analysis you have to choose the solutions that work for you.

- **Choose for the future, but only the future you understand.** Don't be seduced by other people's visions. What matters is the one you and your colleagues create for your system.

- **Use off-the-shelf solutions wherever you can.** It's cheaper and easier to update, as you certainly will have to over time.

- **Pick solutions that are flexible and compatible with your other systems.** You are building a network of IT capabilities. They have to talk to each other, and equally important, the data needs to be as compatible as possible for purposes of aggregation.

- **Minimize customization as you implement,** as it costs more, lengthens the rollout phase, slows upgrades, and makes them more expensive when you do them. The more you customize, the more likely it is that individual systems will be incompatible.

- **Do whatever homework and data cleanup is necessary before you implement.** Don't wait until after the new system is in place to do it; too hard, too long, too much garbage.

- **Plan your rollout carefully.** Invest adequately in the people and resources to do it right. And be patient.

- **Budget generously for system maintenance and upgrades.** The rule of thumb is that for every dollar spent to buy and implement a system, you need to budget at least an equivalent amount for maintenance and upgrades. Systems generally require upgrades every few years. The price of these varies, but it is essential to build them into your projections. Don't delay the upgrades; they get more expensive the longer you wait.

To lead these efforts, you will need a central decision group (an IT Steering Committee, for example) made up of respected thought leaders and clinicians, as well as outside experts and, above all, patients. The group should oversee the design and implementation of your information system. They should recommend policy for data definitions, privacy, customization, and diligence; screen and recommend specific IT solutions; oversee their implementation; review and decide on customization requests; ensure data compatibility; and oversee the analytic function. The group is your partner in developing the overall Information System Plan, and they are accountable to you, the board, and the organization for ensuring its success.

Your information system is a key requirement for delivering superior care in the twenty-first century. Your technology infrastructure makes it possible to collect, distribute, and use the information. To build that infrastructure effectively, you need agreement about what it must do, and a strategy for how and in what order to build it. Otherwise your approach will be random and unnecessarily expensive, the infrastructure will not fit together, and the synergies you must have will not happen. As you develop your plans, you should keep in mind simple guidelines to ensure that you build the system you need, do not overspend doing it, and have what you need soon enough to be helpful in the transformation you have begun.

CHAPTER EIGHTEEN

PRODS

The status quo is a powerful magnet, and prods help you escape its pull. Like the "picador" in the Spanish bullfight, prods are designed to provoke the organization to do what may be difficult, weaken its resistance to change, and forestall the tendency to return to the past. Four are particularly useful. First are institutes that operate at right angles to the organization. Second are outside consultants who can help the organization move from one point to the next at crucial times in the change journey. Third are other visiting experts, individuals who provide useful insights for the organization, and whose reputations lend weight to these observations. Last are the internal consultants whose participation helps people identify better ways to provide care, evaluate these improvements, and make further modifications again and again.

INSTITUTES

An institute has no ongoing operational responsibilities; its purpose is to help those who do focus on the improvement and innovation agendas of the organization. Entities like these can address a range of issues. For example, the Care Management Institute (CMI) at Kaiser Permanente introduces new information about clinical care and helps the practitioners incorporate these advances into their daily practices. The Lean Institutes at Virginia Mason and ThedaCare provide training in that quality improvement method, while the Center for Urban Studies at Mt. Sinai in Chicago helps study and organize the communities served by the institution to address health-related issues, including accessing appropriate and timely medical care. At Long Island Hospitals, the Education Center trains all employees, including physicians, in the purposes, approaches, and values of the organization. It is also the location for the new medical school designed to prepare physicians for collaborative practice in medical homes. While these differ in focus, they have several characteristics in common:

Characteristics

These institutes are funded as a separate line item in the annual operating budget of the organization or system. These operating funds support the people and systems needed to carry out the mission, and are committed for the long term depending on results (see below). Because these institutes are part of the larger strategy, similar to the innovation program, they are treated as strategic investments. Only in the worst circumstances would leaders reduce the funding for reasons unrelated to performance. Their purpose is to influence and provoke the operations, but they do not become enmeshed in the daily challenges and responsibilities of providing care for patients. They are led by credible senior people, and governed by a board that reports directly to the CEO and the board of directors of the parent institution. They have hire and fire power over their staff as long as they follow the policies, rules and regulations that guide the larger system, and they usually rely on support services from the parent organization to minimize their overhead. If the focus is clinical, the institute can be located in the physician organization. Otherwise it is part of the system itself. Depending on the particular mission of the institute, it is free to develop outside funding sources that supplement the mission. Finally, and critically important, the mission is explicit, the expectations are clear, and the oversight is as rigorous as for all other parts of the organization.

The role of the institute is to provide expertise and a consistent and independent perspective on how well and how fast the system is changing. Functioning properly, it forces the organization to do better, helps it stay focused, and plays a key role in encouraging the organization to learn. It must be independent yet serve the interests and needs of the larger organization. It has to walk a fine line between provoking and standing back, criticizing and helping, as well as developing independent solutions and building on those that emerge from within the organization. It must resist the temptation to engage in operations, even when those in operations stand back or seek to shift responsibility to the institute. It is always the picador, not the matador. In the press of daily business, it is the "truth teller," a trusted independent voice about how things should be done, what things are worth doing, and whose voices are important to hear.

Examples

The Care Management Institute (CMI) at Kaiser Permanente. The CMI, started in 1997, has two purposes: (1) to build evidence-based approaches to diagnosis and treatment of key clinical problems that carry significant morbidity and mortality for patients and consume substantial resources of the organization; and (2) develop and implement tools that help clinicians incorporate these approaches into their daily practices. In addition the CMI tracks the diffusion of their efforts. A similar role is played by the Institute for Clinical Systems Improvement (ICSI), a large Minnesota collaborative begun in 1963.

Since its inception, the CMI has built an extensive diffusion infrastructure made up of physician thought leaders, each of whom is paired with a non-physician educator partner. These leaders help individual physicians and other clinicians change their practices to conform with the evidence-based approaches, a process that is particularly difficult because it involves helping individual clinicians change deeply ingrained habits. Knowledge is part of the solution, of course, but learning new ways to dance, in effect, is the most crucial and difficult challenge of all.

The CMI is led by a physician chosen by its independent board of directors made up of eight representatives from the Permanente Medical Groups and two from the Kaiser Foundation Health Plan and Hospitals organization, working in collaboration with the Permanente Federation. The expert committees who review the evidence and develop the content include clinical experts from within and outside the organization. Staff support focuses on data discovery, analysis, and synthesis under the direction of the expert committees.

The success of CMI is a result of its focus on clinical problems that affect the lives of many patients, its relentless efforts to diffuse the knowledge into daily practice, and its rigor. Importantly, it is a creature of the physician groups. The Health Plan and Hospitals organization provides funding and receives an annual update of progress toward the stipulated objectives of knowledge creation and diffusion. But the CMI is "owned" by the physicians. The long process to implement an EMR solution throughout the organization was built on the content produced by the CMI, incorporating CMI guidelines into its decision support modules to reinforce the diffusion efforts.

The CMI has evolved significantly over its 15-year history. Today, for example, its experts work side by side with patients in the design of care pathways and delivery solutions. Throughout its history, it has played an important catalytic role at Kaiser Permanente. At the time of its creation, most of the twelve independent medical groups sponsored their own content-creation efforts, producing practice recommendations that sometimes overlapped but were often in conflict. The quality of the work varied too, as did efforts to diffuse the content into practice. This is no longer the case thanks to the persistence and success of CMI. There is far greater willingness to find shared solutions across the regions and independent medical groups. And the products of the CMI are the gold standard for the organization, drawing on the expertise of clinicians from across the Program.

The CMI was created despite the skepticism of many of the physician leaders. They eventually supported it because it was under their collective control through its board of directors and the Permanente Federation. Even then some physician leaders continued to fund their independent content-development efforts until the rigor of the CMI and the inclusiveness of the effort carried the day. For the most part, the individual Permanente medical groups are satisfied now with the content-creation efforts of the CMI, and work closely with the CMI to diffuse the clinical strategies in their individual medical groups.

The Virginia Mason Institute. Virginia Mason leaders, like those at ThedaCare in Wisconsin and Intermountain Healthcare in Utah, have established an institute to train its people, as well as others who wish to learn the method the organization embraces to achieve the significant transformation in its care quality and efficiency. This entity is the keeper of the method. It includes experts in the Virginia Mason adaptation of the Toyota Lean production system and management system. Its staff help coordinate the annual visit by board members, senior leaders, thought leaders, managers, and select staff to attend the two week training program arranged by Shingijutsu, former Toyota engineers, in Japan. And most importantly, it ensures that the organization stays true to its commitment to the method, utilizing the appropriate rigor in its application of the method and tools.

The Center for Public Health (Mt. Sinai Hospital and Medical Center, Chicago, Illinois). This is a different kind of institute. Its goal is to organize leaders and members of local communities around efforts to measure, then address the root causes of their illness burdens. It receives some funding from Mt. Sinai, supplemented with grants and contracts from local and state public health entities, as well as federal sources. Although it has had some impact on patterns of illness, it remains a work in progress. Moreover, there has been little impact thus far on the medical delivery system. For the most part, the efforts have focused outward, away from the medical care system. Bridges between the community programs and the care system are still limited. Longer term, however, the leaders of the institute realize that their impact will grow substantially if they can use the community organizations they've created to work with the medical care system and providers to find more seamless ways for patients to move back and forth between the care system and their homes and communities.

When you are enmeshed in the daily challenges of running your organization, it's often hard to step back, to stay focused on the larger goals, and remain loyal to the larger purposes and values. You will be pressured to compromise, just a little here, then there, until pretty soon you're off course. An institute can help you avoid this trap. It reminds you why you are doing things the way you are, and why they are important to your long-term mission. It reinforces the methods you have chosen even when they are onerous, or appear irrelevant to the immediate problem at hand.

One can lead without an institute, of course. It isn't as essential as a collaborative medical staff or a committed work force or a supportive board of directors. But without the institute the job of changing the organization is harder. It is a tool that can help you achieve what you seek, and without it you have to spend more energy to keep the organization on track. You're never free of that responsibility, of course, but the institute, properly constituted and funded, can help you move faster and in a more focused way than you might otherwise be able to.

OUTSIDE CONSULTANTS

Used well, outside consultants provide valuable perspectives and helpful expertise. Used poorly, however, they are an unnecessary expense and bring unwanted disruptions to the transformation process. If you view them as "prods" to help you keep the organization moving, or to get it started again when the change process stalls, you will use them most effectively. They should not become permanent fixtures, nor should they take on work best done by people within the organization. Sometimes, however, the situation requires a longer engagement, and in special circumstances, you may need to have outsiders carrying out specific work that would normally be done inside. But generally, outside consultants have the greatest impact when they are retained to do specific work, or to provoke the organization at a crucial point.

Consultants, of course, are not all created equal. Their effectiveness varies considerably from person to person. When you are using outsiders to do work that the organization cannot do (supplement the financial operations, carry out audits, provide industrial engineering expertise, etc.), skills and expertise are more important than consulting experience and effectiveness. But when outsiders are brought in to prod the organization ahead, they must have the necessary gravitas to influence the organization as you intend them to.

Because consultants are often expensive, usually far more so than the costs of employing people in the organization, there can be a temptation to bring people in "on the cheap": hire less expensive consultants; dicker over nickels and dimes; or narrow the scope of work; etc. This is penny-wise and pound-foolish; you get what you pay for. If you're lucky, you may run across an individual or a firm who is unusually inexpensive and effective. This is an exception, though, a very small needle in a very large haystack. Your time is better spent finding a consultant you respect who is backed by a strong firm with a solid reputation. You want to make sure others the consultant brings with her can do the job too. And you want to negotiate a reasonable scope of work for a fair price to both parties, then concentrate on getting the value from the consultation rather than spending time on the bills and charges and specific "deliverables."

Consultants need room to maneuver and freedom to prod effectively. Their value grows as they listen and learn, and as they share their insights as they progress. Sometimes you will want their views on a specific matter, a particular initiative, or a new strategic direction. More often, though, you need them to provide a yardstick to help you calibrate how your changes are progressing and where more work is needed to keep them in place or get them back on track. If the consultant is hired to produce an opinion on a specific matter, the scope of work and the deliverables should reflect this. But if she has been brought in to calibrate and advise, you want a broader scope of work unencumbered by unneeded, usually inappropriate details. In these circumstances you should agree ahead of time that the engagement will continue only as long as you get value from it. All engagements should have a specific end date. These can be modified if necessary, but a value-based, time-bound engagement is most useful for a consultancy directed to helping understand how well the organization is moving forward with its capacity-building efforts.

You can also use outside consultants to deliver unwelcome or difficult news. At certain points in a major change process, this can be quite helpful, especially when the alternative is for you or someone in the organization to do it and pay the price politically that is sure to result. Good consultants are used to being lightning rods; it comes with the territory. If selected wisely, properly oriented to the issues you face, and given the opportunity to listen and learn from others, a consultant can be exactly what you need to break through the logjam. Maturity and experience are prerequisites for credibility to address these kinds of problems and deliver tough messages. You don't want to constrain the consultant unnecessarily in a situation like this, although you certainly want to resist the pressure you may receive from her to help you take further steps once the messages have been delivered.

Finally, it is crucial to stay connected to your outside consultants. You need to meet with them regularly, debrief often, and interact and direct them to ensure they don't get off track. This level of involvement is the key to effective use of outside consultants. You will learn from a good consultant all along the way, you can help the consultant interpret what she hears and learns, and together you can shape the messages and decide how best to deliver them as her conclusions emerge.

OTHER OUTSIDE EXPERTS

In addition to professional consultants, you may want to engage outside experts to review and evaluate different parts of your organization. Many organizations use this approach, especially in higher education, but also in selected healthcare systems. Experts, either individually or as members of small panels, are chosen by leaders of the particular area to be reviewed, or by you and your senior team. They receive comprehensive background information in advance about the department or function; conduct a short, intense visit to see the area firsthand; present their findings and recommendations to the leaders of the target area, the organization, and the board of directors if appropriate; and they may be asked to produce a written summary following the visit that becomes part of the official record for the organization. They may also return to assess progress after a suitable period of time.

While the size of these panels can vary, their makeup is consistent. Members are usually senior professionals who are respected in their field, seasoned in the issues that affect the subject, and recognized for their wisdom and objectivity. They should be people whose words and insights will matter to the people in your organization. Every panel should have a specified scope of work beforehand that is clarified in person by you and other leaders at the outset of the review.

Panels like these are usually paid for their time and related expenses, though they may be persuaded to volunteer if financial constraints are severe. They are treated with respect and dignity, and their findings discussed thoughtfully. The goal for those who receive their reports is not to challenge or debate, but to clarify and understand the findings in order to inform later conversations and actions. The purpose of these efforts, then, is to learn rather than problem solve. The panel must understand, as should all the internal participants, that any recommendations are advisory. Nothing will happen until agreement is reached inside the organization once the findings have been carefully reviewed and evaluated.

You can use panels like these when you have a particular issue to resolve, or a problem department or area that has not made the progress you'd hoped for. You may want experts to validate your approach and provide an outside marker for what you have accomplished. Panels can also become a regular feature of your leadership, used routinely across the organization to review the status on a regular basis throughout the year. They take time to convene and manage, however, so you need to be thoughtful about how many can be managed effectively in the course of a year.

There is an ongoing debate about whether or not to create semi-permanent advisory panels or boards to carry out work like this. You can if this works better for your institution, but there are shortcomings with this approach. With time, standing groups tend to lose their "fresh eyes"—the very insights and reactions that are so valuable to you. They become inured to the shortcomings of the organization, or caught up in the trap of their own process. You have to find ways for them to remain objective and fresh or they aren't worth the effort.

There are several ways to do this. The most dramatic (and expensive) is to bring people in from outside the organization to meet with your advisory panels. These "advisers of the advisers" introduce new ideas—different perspectives in order to stimulate conversations and broaden views. You can regularly change the makeup of the panels themselves, introducing new members who bring different perspectives, setting term limits, and increasing and decreasing the panel sizes from time to time. And you can structure their agendas to challenge assumptions, review data and stories, and ensure that different points of view are heard. You want to be sure there is ample time for conversations within the panels themselves, designed to encourage debate, raise concerns, and challenge you and the leaders of the organization. Show-and-tell meetings that drown the audience in slides and data can stupefy the participants. In fact meetings like this insult them. The purpose of the panels is to hear from *them* not you or your people. They have to know just enough to be helpful, of course, but that can be accomplished with focused preparation and precise presentations.

INSIDE EXPERTS

This is really tricky. You are unlikely to have the industrial engineering, quality improvement, and analytical resources you need to drive your organization forward. Most healthcare organizations don't. If you choose to add them, however, be careful not to overwhelm your operations. You want to have sufficient numbers to keep the organization moving forward, but they have to work side by side with those who do the work, and be selected with care to be sure they have the personalities to consult and advise without trying to control or take over. They must be collaborators who help the teams and groups accomplish their work, not people to whom difficult problems are passed off to so that those doing the work can get back to doing what they prefer.

You do need them though. To assess your delivery system requires people who know how to do these things. Industrial engineers can help design and evaluate production systems. Lean consultants know how to collect and analyze data, establish tolerances, and separate signals from noise, for example. Capable analysts make sense of complex, often confusing data. You need all of them on your team.

As you consider how to build your internal expertise, watch for two traps. The first is most common—money. People with the requisite skills and personalities can be hard to find and expensive. You may be tempted to hire someone less experienced to save costs, but that person will struggle to establish credibility with those who deliver care and will add little value as a result. Or you may be inclined to add these responsibilities to someone already working in the organization, perhaps providing special training to help them carry out this new function. These people can be pulled in multiple directions by competing demands, or function at a level too basic to help. The second trap is the one already mentioned: the temptation for inside consultants to take over an operating area in order to fix it, or the equally pervasive temptation to shift responsibility for enhancing performance or making improvements to the consultants. These temptations arise most commonly when there is controversy or when change becomes difficult. As leader you have to be sure the inside experts do not get trapped this way.

Every organization going through a significant transformation must avoid falling back into the old ways of doing things. Institutes, consultants, outside experts, and inside experts can help you do this. It's hard to do it alone, or to move as far and fast enough as you hope to by relying only on your partners and leadership team. You need more help. Careful use of these prods can help you diminish resistance, get back on course, increase the pace, and above all, remain true to the values and objectives that you have chosen for your future.

CHAPTER NINETEEN

ACCOUNTABILITY AND COMPENSATION

In a gathering of twenty or so people, we puzzled about why it is so difficult to get people to do the right things to make their patients safe. Opinions were evenly divided. One group argued that better incentives were the answer, the other that tighter regulations were required. Paul O'Neill, who served as Secretary of the Treasury under President G.W. Bush, listened for several minutes before offering his views. According to him, the world divides into two camps, those who believe every problem can be solved with money, and those who think laws and regulations are the answer. Neither works very well, at least not alone, O'Neill points out. A challenge like this requires both, combined in a thoughtful and comprehensive program. The same is true when it comes to an accountability and compensation system for your organization.

Your accountability and compensation system is another important lever to help you communicate and reinforce key values and strategies of the organization. In addition, it enables you to attract and retain a high-quality workforce, and reward people for exceptional work that furthers the agenda of the organization. Several principles should guide you as you develop your program.

First and foremost, this is *your* system; you have to design it to work for what you want to accomplish. There is no "right" way to do it. You can learn from others, of course, but your solution has to reflect *your* needs and realities. Even if you delegate its day-to-day administration, the design decisions must remain up to you. You need to keep a close eye on how it works in practice to adjust and improve it with experience. Especially early in your tenure, it is imperative to control both elements of the program to be sure people know what they are expected to do and are rewarded for the things you, your board, and your leadership team have agreed should be recognized. Because these elements send such powerful messages throughout the organization about what is "really" important, your program is an essential part of the language you use to shape perceptions and drive performance.

Second, change your system carefully. Although you may want to evaluate and modify it as you gain experience, keep in mind a special caution as you do. To communicate a clear and consistent message about the values at the heart of the organization and the performance levers for building the capabilities you seek requires steady, relentless effort. You can change your messages and the tools you use to reinforce them, but only with careful planning. In my experience it takes a year or two at least, and often longer, before people begin to understand their accountabilities and how they will be rewarded, no matter how simple and clear your program may be. You have to explain it again and again. A useful rule of thumb is to leave your system in place for three to four years before you modify it in any significant way, and then expect to spend another year or two explaining why you want to change it and what you hope to accomplish.

Third, emphasize teams and groups, not individuals. The most striking shift required to create your new culture is from the individualistic, hierarchical model of today to a flatter, coordinated, team-based delivery system in which outstanding care is delivered through successful collaboration across specialties, professional boundaries, organizational levels, and the individuals and groups your organization serves. Accountabilities and compensation should reward team and group performance and results instead of individual contributions and effort. If you can, you want to shift responsibility for meeting expectations and for dividing the rewards for excellent performance to the team or group. This may seem to be an abrogation of responsibility, but in fact it is a powerful tool to achieve compliance with expected norms and performance.

Fourth, you want to emphasize mission, values, and operating principles in your accountability and rewards system. The care system you anticipate requires three things of every person: outstanding performance in delivering or supporting the delivery of care; consistency with the values of the organization; and collaboration with colleagues and patients (and communities when appropriate) to find better ways to deliver and improve care. When someone is new in her job, you may need to detail specific accountabilities, and the promotion, pay, and reward opportunities that occur as a result of meeting them. After an appropriate period of time, however, the accountabilities and rewards should begin to reflect the central purposes that every person in the organization must fulfill. Overly detailed accountabilities and rewards systems can inhibit the performance you want to develop. You will want to have unambiguous boundary expectations for the three areas, but within those broad boundaries, you want to encourage individual and team creativity and innovation.

Fifth, an accountability and compensation system based on this principle of boundaries requires coaching and feedback. Your people need help to understand where the boundaries lie, how to interpret them, and how to focus their time in order to develop improved ways to do their work. This immediate, collaborative learning helps create the environment you need by reinforcing the principles of respect and collaboration, and encouraging people to act in the best interests of the organization. There must be a limit to your tolerance. When someone fails to improve with coaching, or displays willful disregard of the values of the organization, you have to act. There can be no ambiguity. Ideally everyone will know why you are taking the action. Your actions to define what the boundaries are and what it means when they are ignored or violated communicate loudly and help refine the meaning of those boundaries as well.

Common wisdom dictates that detailed accountabilities (e.g. Management by Objectives, or MBO-based pay) and individualized compensation and rewards are required to get top performance. I don't agree. Detailed accountabilities force individuals to focus on compliance instead of identifying, testing, and improving new care delivery solutions. Similarly, individual incentives and rewards reinforce individual achievement rather than collaboration. The power of individual incentives decays with time as well. You have to keep raising the ante for the individual incentives to reinforce what you wish. If you don't, the incentives (or "at risk" compensation) become an expected part of compensation.

It may not be possible to do away with individual incentives completely. After all, this approach is part of the fabric of most organizational and corporate compensation programs in the United States at least. People may be lured away by hefty individual compensation programs and arrangements that you have difficulty matching. Be careful how you respond, however. Individual rewards are "loud" in terms of the message they communicate through the organization. People usually know who has been singled out, and they interpret the stories about any special individual reward you might offer through the deeply ingrained filters so characteristic of organizational cultures. You can undo a lot of work in a short period of time with ill-timed or ill-conceived individual rewards. Trying to match offers from competitors in order to retain a high performer is also a slippery slope. It is hard to know where to stop, where the moment comes to wish the person good luck and stop modifying your principles to retain her.

With these general considerations in mind, I'd offer the following specific recommendations for the compensation portion of your program.

A Suggested Compensation Program

There are as many compensation programs as compensation consultants and organizations. Each is a variation on basic themes, however, and the overarching principles are similar.

Definitions. An important challenge is to define what you mean by compensation. Typically compensation refers to base salary, "at risk" income that depends on performance, and the benefits provided by the organization. Total compensation is the sum of these elements. At risk income can include annual and longer-term bonuses linked to the achievement of target performance levels. As mentioned these are most effective when delivered in the context of group or team performance, and to the performance of the organization as a whole. Benefits can take many forms, ranging from a collection of specific benefits to a benefit "pool" in the form of a cash payment to individuals to use to purchase prescribed benefits.

Structure. Your system should be easy to administer and understand. Fewer pay "bands" are helpful—between five and six altogether—with variations within each band based on assessments of performance. These variations should respond to issues of internal equity, so that as people learn about one another's compensation, they see few obvious differences except those related to measured performance. Gender and ethnic differences, and rewards for longevity without consideration of performance have no place in an equitable compensation program.

To establish your compensation ranges, including benefit structures, you need an appropriate comparator group. Although examples may be difficult to find, you should try to construct a comparator group of thirty to fifty organizations to minimize idiosyncratic, year-to-year variations. It can also be helpful to identify three to five systems whose pay practices you admire, and use them as a qualitative check on the numbers and pay practices obtained from the larger comparator group. Whatever comparator process you choose, try to keep it simple, understandable, predictable and as stable as you can for as long as you can.

Management. You want to work with your board to establish the parameters of your compensation program, review and approve it in detail, and ratify the results for year-to-year compensation and rewards adjustments. The board should use the same parameters to set your compensation. You and your senior team should establish the parameters and review the results each year to ensure that your program is applied as intended.

Incentives. As mentioned, the incentive program of the organization should emphasize team, group, and department results. It should be the responsibility of each cluster to recommend how to divide the rewards among its members. They should be coached in how to do this to be consistent with the priorities of the organization. Depending on the size of your organization, you may want to delegate the approval authority to different leaders, but the overall program, and particularly the decisions about key areas of the organization should remain with you; your role in overseeing the system should be unambiguous.

You may wish to reserve a pool of money to reward special efforts and unexpectedly good results. These may be directed to teams and groups, but you can also use such awards for individuals in unusual circumstances. The key is to make the recognition more about what the individual achieved than the amount of money she earned. You want it to be significant enough that the individual and the people of the organization see it as serious, but you also want to emphasize why the special grant has been made in the context of the transformation underway. These awards should be granted irregularly and infrequently to be "special." It is always important to link them to the organizational strategies and values to avoid undermining the critical focus on collaboration to drive the organization forward.

Cash vs. Non-cash Rewards. The combination of cash and non-cash awards is powerful in reinforcing key priorities and values. Cash rewards can be placed in a pool to divide among the members of teams, groups, or departments, or can be an award to the cluster itself to enhance staffing, buy special equipment, pay for a dinner for the team, etc. You can do both. And you can also use recognition events, non-cash rewards such as restaurant gift certificates, vacation rewards, and the like, to further honor group achievement. The larger the event at which these awards are announced, the more broadly you can broadcast why they have been given. There is also a place for quiet awards, ones not publicized. These, too, should reflect performance focused on key priorities. Here you must rely on the informal grapevine to communicate your decision, but this too can send strong signals about the behaviors that are important.

Longevity vs. Performance. I've mentioned already my preference for performance-based awards over those for longevity. But there is a place for rewarding loyalty and the steadfastness that longevity represents with non-cash recognition ceremonies and rewards. These can highlight the contributions of the people in the organization who by their longevity are often the backbone of the place even though they may not be high-flying superstars and opinion leaders. You know who they are and what they do for patients day in and day out. You know too that not all are outstanding, and not all make great or consistent contributions to their teams or departments. But they are people who matter, and the fact that you recognize them for their commitment to the organization sends yet another important message about respect for everyone's contributions.

Profit Sharing. Sharing profits is a powerful tool to create a sense of collective responsibility. This can be tricky in a 501(c)(3) organization that doesn't have "profits" in the sense that a for-profit entity does. It is also tricky when your organization has union contracts to negotiate. But if you can work through these barriers, you will be well served to establish such a program. In the case of a not-for-profit entity, you can designate a profit pool to be paid only after all other obligations have been met and the residual (retained) earnings cover longer term capital costs. A similar arrangement can be made in a for-profit institution. Payments in this instance are usually made to individuals. How you distribute the payments is your choice: a single sum for each person, a specific sum for everyone in a particular compensation band, a percent-age of total annual cash compensation, etc. To be effective, the pro-gram should represent a significant source of income, link directly to overall organizational performance, and vary significantly with the year-to-year results. It is conceivable to link profit sharing and groups and teams by distributing the shares to them and letting them decide how to divide them further among the individual participants. I have not seen this in practice, however, and cannot suggest that you do it based on my personal experience.

One important issue in the design of a profit sharing program is whether or not it should be an all-or-nothing pool or awarded in proportion to the financial results. I favor the latter. For example, if the total pool is $1 million when financial performance (profits) reaches the targeted levels, it should be some percentage of that total if the profits reach only 75 percent of the target. With each increment above 75 percent in profits, the pool fills correspondingly until it is full at the target. If profits exceed target, you may wish to share the upside as well. You will want to cap the total at 125 percent or so to prevent unforeseen windfalls that could distort expectations and the long-term objectives you have established. As described below, an incentive program linked to financial performance must have an all-or-nothing quality gate in order to reinforce the course you are pursuing.

The Quality Gate. If you don't meet your quality targets as an organization or part of an organization, no profits should be shared. The last message you want to send to your patients, your organization and the community is that people in your organization have been rewarded financially when performing below your quality standards and objectives. Imagine how patients and the community will respond if you make profit sharing payments to everyone in the organization in a year that you fail to meet your safety objectives, in a year people died or were harmed by errors you can prevent. This is political suicide for a not-for-profit organization, and creates serious credibility problems for for-profit institutions as well. With a transparent organization, there is no question about what these standards are, who has set them, and to whom they apply. Similarly, there should be no question about why people in the organization have earned or failed to earn their incentive payments, whatever the form those payments might take.

Traps

There are three traps to avoid in any accountability and compensation system. First is the exception or the special deal. This is death in an organization unless it furthers the larger integration agenda in a way that motivates the organization. Especially troublesome are special deals with individual physicians or with groups of physicians to buy loyalty or business. Sometimes you have no choice; when other institutions try to entice groups of physicians away with large incentive payments and special arrangements, you may have to act to protect your institution. But be careful. Don't get caught in a mini arms race. You may lose some good people because the price of buying their loyalty is too high. So be it. And there are few secrets; once you've agreed to a special arrangement, most of the physicians on your medical staff will know about it, and others will as well. You will certainly come under pressure to do the same or more for the next group or individual physician. Once that happens, the ball never stops rolling.

The second trap is the belief that money is the answer. Don't underestimate the power of your culture, of belonging and familiarity. Don't hesitate to use non-monetary enticements to motivate and retain your workforce, once you are convinced that the monetary rewards you provide are fair. Opportunities to serve on leadership teams, receive special training, participate on innovation projects, and lead improvement projects can create strong bonds. Recognition for outstanding work does too, especially in the context of what teams and groups and departments have accomplished. Colleagueship is critically important; if people develop strong ties to the people they work with, they are less likely to leave, even when the package may be potentially more generous.

The final trap is the water torture approach to addressing hiring and retention problems. It is tempting when someone is offered a strong package to move to another organization to create a "just good enough" response. It is a variant on the "just this once" phenomenon. Like most leaders, you are a pragmatist. You often can solve a problem with a tweak or minor modification. But you have to be careful. You want to avoid adjustments that force you to modify your basic compensation strategy. If you can adjust the base salary by a few percentage points to finalize an agreement for someone to join the organization, that might be acceptable. If, on the other hand, it becomes necessary to strike a deal that you make with no other person, it violates your compensation principles and should be avoided. Incremental changes to retain someone or some group may appear innocent one by one, but together they may subvert your basic philosophy.

You cannot prevent someone who wants to leave from doing so, and the story often turns out poorly when you do. But you can build strong bonds between the individual and your institution that help you retain the people you want: the way you work as colleagues, and the fairness and comprehensiveness of the way you create expectations and compensate people. Troubles arise when the measuring stick in an organization is weighted too far towards the financial rewards at the expense of the host of non-financial rewards and connections that create a fulfilling professional and employment experience. And trouble also arises when you make incremental modifications to your program in order to accommodate individual demands, and slowly undermine the integrity of what you have created as a result.

Your accountability and compensation program is the final system you must put in place to drive your organization on its new course. It is tempting to over-engineer it, to dampen creativity and initiative by being too specific about accountabilities and too precise in compensation opportunities. To deliver outstanding care requires cooperation, teamwork and collaboration. Both the accountabilities you establish and the rewards you provide must reinforce these behaviors. Moreover the rewards you provide—in whatever form—should depend entirely on whether or not the organization and its elements meet all quality expectations. Without this focus, the many efforts you make to establish this direction can be for naught. You confuse the organization and those who depend on it.

CHAPTER TWENTY

OPERATING DISCIPLINE

You have identified the building blocks you need to establish the three complementary operations required to provide the best care possible: delivery excellence, discovery, and improvement. How do you decide what to work on first? How do you set your priorities? How can you be sure these operations work as intended to propel the organization forward?

In information technology an operating system organizes and controls hardware and software so that the device it lives in behaves in a flexible but predictable way. Without it there is chaos, a mishmash of data and algorithms and electronics that don't fit together. The same is true for your organization. To achieve its purposes and goals requires a powerful discipline that enables you to organize and shape the hardware (systems, physical resources) and software (in our case, people) to behave in a "...flexible but predictable way." Without it you are left with individual professionalism and hope, and a high probability that you will make little headway in improving your performance. What are the characteristics of such a discipline?

The place to start is to examine how different organizations have achieved uncommon results. How does Virginia Mason reduce the time from back injury to return to work? How does ThedaCare drive the door-to-balloon time down so far? How does Denver Health achieve number one ranking among its peer hospital systems in Colorado, or rank first among academic medical centers in the country for observed versus expected Medicare mortality rates? How has Intermountain Healthcare achieved such substantial improvements in quality and still drive down costs? How did Norton Health win its recent award for quality? How did the North Shore-Long Island Jewish Health System create its culture of patient centeredness? How does Cincinnati Children's Hospital achieve its uncommon outcomes for children? How can Kaiser Permanente members experience lower rates of cardiac illness than any other group, reduced mortality from colon cancer, and virtually no hospitalizations for children with asthma? What do these organizations have in common?

They and many others have an explicit discipline for how they get things done, a well-developed operating system. Virginia Mason leaders even call theirs the Virginia Mason Operating System. John Toussaint, MD, the CEO of ThedaCare who began the transformation of that organization and now leads their institute, has written two books about the approach they have used to transform the care they provide. They may differ from one to the next, but these operating disciplines share certain characteristics:

They are up to the challenge. These approaches are robust, rigorous and tough-minded. They have produced excellent results consistent with their respective purposes. And they have done so over an extended period of time. They have proven their worth.

They reinforce the systems required to deliver the best care possible consistent with the underlying values the organizations have agreed to. These organizations have chosen their discipline to match and reinforce their goals and values. The operating system is not peripheral, an add-on, a toolbox applied here and there; the discipline is central to how they do business and how they work.

They are teachable and reproducible. An operating system is of little consequence if only a few use it, or if those who do use it as they choose. Every one of the organizations mentioned uses their operating system all the time, everywhere. It is how they do their business. Everyone is expected to learn what the discipline is, what it involves, what the rules are, and what the tools are.

They are analytical and data driven and complement patient stories and expectations. These organizations know that to deliver the best care possible requires a clear understanding of what is done. Care cannot be changed, improved, reassessed, changed again, further perfected, redesigned, or re-invented unless it is measured. Their discipline is rooted in numbers, measurement, data, and given meaning by patient and provider stories and insights. Their mantra is "prove it so we can get better."

They focus on the day-to-day work everyone does. These organizations know that the operating discipline must be applied at every level of the organization by the people who do the work. Everyone needs it to know what she does now, how to make it better, and whether or not she has done so. Everyone needs to know the expectations and be able to use the tools in order to meet them. This approach is workforce driven not expert driven. In some organizations, experts reinforce the discipline and support the improvement and innovation efforts, but they do not do the work.

One, not many. Each of these organizations has made a bet on one discipline to run their operations. They have avoided the trap of using several that diffuses the discipline and makes the leadership efforts less focused. None choose a discipline centered on internal politics and relationship building per se, although all do this well. The over-riding issue is performance: what it is and how to improve it. The operating system they have chosen brings together the partnerships and systems that enable them to address this issue.

And everyone uses it, including the leaders. The discipline is shared from top to bottom. It is the way their board's operate and expect the entire organization to operate; it is what the leaders do and the way they lead others; it is the way problems are solved and performance measured by everyone, everywhere in the organization.

When change gets hard, or there is intense criticism and push back, it can be seductive to try something else, come at it another way. But it is precisely at times like these that the discipline of a powerful operating system is most crucial. You have to get through the challenges and barriers, and your operating system provides the discipline to do so. The single, common method is essential to achieve a performance transformation of the magnitude you have undertaken.

So which method works best? This is your call. You have to determine what matches your organization's needs. The most rigorous and successful operating discipline over the longest period of time in multiple industries around the world involves some variation on the original Deming quality improvement model. Arguably the most powerful of these is the Lean production model developed by Toyota. Certainly this is the case in healthcare, where a handful of organizations have used the Lean operating system to help transform their performance. Others have achieved significant improvements using variations such as Six Sigma, CQI, and others.

As the leader you depend on multiple levers, building blocks, and partners to accomplish the transformation of your organization. But without the discipline of an appropriate method—a core operating system—you cannot succeed. It is that simple. You will work hard, make changes here and there, and even move the needle on performance somewhat. But you won't change the course your organization is on. You will still make decisions the same way and track the same measures of performance as you have traditionally. Only if you implement a method that is up to the challenges can you build the capacity you need to chart your new course.

CHAPTER TWENTY-ONE

FINAL THOUGHTS

People played different roles on the board of directors of KFHP/H. Bill Foege, for example, was often our healthcare conscience. He has had a storied career in international public health as the architect of the World Health Organization sponsored small pox eradication program that eliminated this disease from the globe; head of the National Centers for Disease Control under the administration of President Carter; head of the Carter Center for many years; and medical advisor to Bill and Melinda Gates during the formative years of the Gates Foundation. He chooses words and stories carefully and has the unique perspective of a clinician and public health leader who has been part of healthcare for several decades. When he spoke, we listened closely.

In a series of meetings, the board considered how fast to improve the safety of care for our patients and members. There was no doubt about our commitment. Our concerns were with money and what we could manage: how much to invest and how much time to devote given the many pressing matters that we were dealing with at the time. Foege asked a few questions and then, near the end of the discussions, offered this observation.

"For me it is a simple matter." He said. *"When our members are harmed or die from medical errors we know how to prevent, we are complicit in every injury and every death that occurs until we can stop them from happening."*

Complicity, he argued, is a well-established legal principle and a powerful moral construct. We are responsible for what happens because we know better. Foege reframed the issue. How long, he asked, were we willing to allow our members to suffer harm and death that we knew how to prevent? How long were we willing to be morally and legally wrong? Instead of deciding among equally important priorities, Foege demanded that we do what is right, then figure out how to make it happen as fast as possible.

Complicity is an important idea. It applies to patient safety: when we fail to provide care as safely as we know how. And it applies more broadly to the quality of our care as well: when we knowingly provide care that doesn't work or is ineffective, when we are insensitive and unresponsive, when we waste resources we know how to conserve, or when we fail to treat patients equally because they come from different backgrounds. We are complicit because these are potentially harmful choices that we know how to prevent. We know how to find or discover the best care possible, and when we fail to do so, when we fail to lead our organizations toward this goal, we are responsible for the harm that we inflict as a result.

Throughout this book, I've argued that this is the most powerful reason to make superior quality your destination. It is the right thing to do. As the leader of your organization you have promised you will deliver the safest, most effective, responsive, timely, efficient, and equitable care you can discover or invent—whatever its source—to improve the health of your patients, lower the costs of their care, and improve the health of the communities that depend on you. This is the destination you set out for, to deliver the best care possible to every patient and all patients, every time, all the time. Because of the nature of our science, the technologies at our disposal, and the diversity of our patients and their illnesses, we can always learn more, we can always improve. So you will never arrive. Your journey is the important thing, then, your continuous discovery, your unending search to meet the needs of each person you serve.

Choosing this destination is not only a moral choice. Pursuit of superior quality also provides the two important pillars you need to compete effectively: the trust of your patients and communities, and efficiency with which you operate. As I've argued again and again throughout this book, it is hard to convince people to use your services when they don't trust you, and especially challenging when they have another choice. Trust is an elusive gift that depends on many things you do. Of those, quality is the most important, that elusive mix of the safety, effectiveness, responsiveness, timeliness, efficiency, and equity of the care you provide them.

To deliver care this way requires that you make care simpler, the care processes more easily navigated and reliable, more transparent, so the patient can move from start to finish more easily without wasted time. And this means the care is more efficient and less costly, because when the care processes are engineered to provide reliable, predictable, and straight-forward care like this, you eliminate the lost, repeated, and confusing work that exists everywhere in healthcare. This is the most powerful way to reduce your operating costs. Of course you can reduce your unit costs by cutting staff, or negotiating a discount for a new technology, or by holding the line on raises. But these rarely deliver the ongoing savings you need to be competitive, and they often end up compromising your ability to deliver what your patients want. There are far better ways to obtain the savings that generate the margins to support your future in a world of shrinking payments.

As you look ahead the future looks stormy. We cannot predict with certainty what it will bring, nor is there any action that can eliminate all risks. No matter what we do, how many capabilities we put in place, how wise and experienced we are as leaders, we always must acknowledge the possibility that events may overtake us. Just like what happened to the Columbia Trader in the storm off the coast of the Aleutian Islands.

But the answer is not to throw up our hands and do nothing, or hunker down and hope that what we've always done will protect us from what we cannot know. There is a wiser course. In 1995, David Nadler and his colleagues observed that the companies that tried new things, learned, and adapted, were more likely to survive periods of disruptive change than those following their traditional course. Doing what you've always done doesn't provide much protection when the future is uncertain. Although you can narrow the range of futures to consider through a scenario-planning process, for example, there is no way to be certain. We guess and hope, but only the lucky are right. So what matters is your ability to learn and experiment at a pace that matches the demands of the world you live in, your flexibility and responsiveness, and the capacity you build to help you adapt and change with new information and insights.

This is what the pursuit of superior quality gives you, this journey of discovery and change, and continuous improvement. Your quality journey gives you the best chance of emerging from the storms we are in now and those that lie ahead. Because when you prepare yourself to lead, build the resilient partnerships and systems you need, and establish the operating discipline you must have to integrate these tools that drive your organization forward, you have put in place the capabilities you need to protect your organization in the future. To provide superior care to the patient who appears today requires the same organizational capabilities you need to provide superior care tomorrow...the same ability to discover or invent what works best, then make it better and better.

This is what sets you apart as a leader. Not position or prestige, kudos or financial rewards. It is how well you set this course, and how effectively you build your capacity to follow it successfully. It is how seriously and honestly you explore who you are and what you believe, and how you choose to lead. It is how you establish your presence in the organization and how you build your relationships over time. It is how you prepare the organization to continue the journey long after you step aside. It is how well you can build the partnership you need with those around you, especially with the patients and communities you serve. It is how robust the systems are that you establish to help you steer the organization forward: the systems of language, learning, transparency, information, innovation, prods, and accountability and compensation. And finally it is how well you use an operating discipline to integrate these capabilities into a coherent force to change the course you are on now.

This is your challenge. Not to get better within the narrow confines of business as usual, but to identify the course you want to pursue, and to help those in the organization leave behind the comfort of what they know to join you on this journey without end. It is a difficult, challenging leadership task, not without risks for you and those around you. But the alternatives are riskier. In healthcare it is always preferable to do the right thing. When doing so also provides greater competitive strength and financial well-being, and at the same time, greater likelihood of success in the longer term, there is really no other responsible choice. In my mind, the highest risk option you have is to continue what you've always done, to opt for the comfort of the known at the expense of delivering the best care possible. Your imperative as a leader is to leave your organization stronger than you found it. Hopefully this guide provides you a way to do so.

APPENDIX A:
RECOMMENDATIONS
by CHAPTER

PART ONE – **PREPARING TO LEAD**

WHY CHANGE? (Chapter One)
Because the current systems suffer from:
1. Inconsistent quality
2. Uncertain competitive and financial capabilities
3. Inflexibility to respond to future challenges

WHAT DOES THE NEW ORGANIZATION LOOK LIKE? (Chapter Two)
1. Bridges
2. Process
3. Collaboration
4. Speed
5. Coherence and Constancy

HOW DO YOU LEAD? (Chapter Three)
1. Strong moral core
2. Personal awareness
3. Humanity and compassion
4. Constant study
5. Interest in learning
6. Strong, complementary people
7. Deep presence and involvement throughout organization
8. Shared work
9. Independence
10. Flexibility
11. Sense of timing and possibility
12. Ability to generate engagement and creativity

STARTING (Chapter Four)

    A. Purpose: break with the past and establish strong informal power system

    B. Characteristics

        1. Use initial months to break with the past

        2. Establish informal power system

            Time

            Targets

            Process

        3. Delay decisions

        4. Learn from the people of the organization

        5. Begin succession plan

        6. Set resignation date

OBSTACLES AND TRAPS (Chapter Five)

    A. Obstacles

        1. Financial

            Invest up front

            Find least damaging pilots

            Focus on bundled payments, contracts, prepaid arrangements

            Seek special arrangements with employers

            Establish innovation funds

            Seek support from foundations and community sources

        2. Legal and Regulatory

            Contract or hire specialist in health law

        3. Bandwidth

            Learn from others

            Invest in needed resources

    B. Traps

        1. Bubble Boy

        2. Shiny Objects

        3. Hubris

        4. Kumbaya Decision-making

        5. I'm Owed

YOUR HEALTH (Chapter Six)

    A. Purpose: maintain your mental, emotional and physical strength, and address your most significant vulnerabilities as a leader

    B. Considerations

        1. Exercise

        2. Diet

        3. Sleep

        4. Alone Time

        5. Family Time

PART TWO – **PARTNERS**

THE HEART OF THE MATTER (Chapter Seven)

A. Purpose: establish an enduring partnership with your most important ally for change

B. Level One: the Patient Care Experience
1. Bill of Rights

    Written and verbal reviews of care options and recommendations for each visit or interaction

    Regular evaluations of all interactions

    All providers trained in expectations for patient engagement and held accountable

2. Ubiquitous Stories

    All scheduled meetings begin with patient story, preferably told by the patient

    Regular newsletter with patient stories and care responses

    Staff recognition for exception patient-centered care

3. Data

    Survey and focus group feedback from patients about their care experience

    Share widely and regularly with clinicians

C. Level Two: Care Design, Improvement, Accountability
1. Teams

    All improvement teams include patients

    Educate patients and team members to work together effectively

    Provide support and regular feedback to reinforce and improve function

2. Surveys and Focus Groups

    Obtain regular patient feedback and insights beyond those provided by members of the teams

D. Level Three: Strategic Planning
1. Include patients, consumers, and community representatives

    Organize planning around specific issues and include two to three patients/consumers/community members on each team

    Roll specific planning efforts into overarching plan to be reviewed by Patient Advisory Council(s) if they exist or in community surveys if not

    Limit strategic priorities to two to three per year and focus on patient care-related matters

E. Level Four: Community Health and Well-Being

    Join with others in communities

Conduct in-depth studies to validate stories and impressions

Support efforts with experts from your institution

Encourage physicians to participate

Invite community leaders to interact with your management teams and board of directors about these efforts and the role of your institution

BOARD OF DIRECTORS (Chapter Eight)

A. Purpose: provide fiduciary and moral stewardship for the organization, and act as your thought partner for the changes underway

B. Considerations

1. Size and Structure

Nine to eleven members optimal

Avoid designated seats if possible

Physicians: only with careful thought

Diverse backgrounds

Predecessor CEO only for defined transition period

2. Contracts and Compacts

Pay retainer and/or charitable match

Define expectations through compact

Conduct regular evaluations of performance

3. Leadership and Terms of Service

Separate CEO and Chairman roles if possible

Establish Board terms with limits on total years served

Evaluate Chairman on same schedule as CEO

4. Meetings

Focus on course change

Start each with patient story

Review performance at every meeting

Include educational component in every meeting if possible

Use standard decision format for all decisions

Five to six scheduled meetings/year optimal; others ad hoc

5. Committee Structure

Simplify fiduciary responsibilities and committees

Establish two strategic committees, Quality and Change Strategy, and assign all members to one or the other

THE SENIOR LEADERSHIP TEAM AND THE CHANGE LEADERSHIP NETWORK (Chapter Nine)

A. Purpose: complement and challenge you, and provide well-rounded skills and perspectives to lead the organization through the changes

B. Senior Leadership Team
  1. Make Up
      Complementary skills and networks to yours
      Mix of perspectives and approaches
      Diversity
  2. Named Positions
      CFO
      HR
      CIO
      All play control/management and strategic roles that are
        central to course change
  3. Dynamics
      Constructive conflict
  4. Organization
      Changes to meet your needs and those of organization
  5. Meetings and Retreats
      Regular and scheduled
      Ad Hoc when needed
      Patient story(ies) always start
      On the floors frequently/regularly
      Routine decision format and preparation discipline
C. Change Leadership Network
      Organic and changing with circumstances
      Groups and individuals

PHYSICIANS (Chapter Ten)

A. Purpose: engage these critical players in the shared search
  for superior quality
B. Considerations
  1. Common Ground
      Patient care and superior quality
  2. Information
      Performance transparency
  3. Exposure to outside solutions
      Regular, hands-on visits to other healthcare and
        non-healthcare entities to learn
  4. Pruning
      Must ask non-performing or obstructionist physicians
        to leave
  5. Organization
      Formal physician organization preferred
  6. Ownership
      Jury out

7. Incentives
    Incentives for group and team performance
    No FFS-like incentives for individual performance

WORKFORCE (Chapter Eleven)

A. Purpose: engage the entire workforce in finding superior care solutions and continuously improving care throughout the organization
B. Considerations
  1. Common Ground
    Patient care and superior quality
  2. Leadership Engagement
    Starting place for workforce engagement
  3. Organizations
    Direct to overall change mission
  4. Unions
    Direct to overall change mission
    Consider formal labor-management partnership
  5. Interest Groups
    Focus on natural affinity groups (African American, Latino, Asian, GLBT, etc.)
    Charter and fund
  6. Story Telling
    Marinate organization in patient stories
    Ubiquitous stories about care giving and care-givers
  7. Fun
    Awards
    Quality
    Safety
    Community Involvement
  8. Retreats and Other Strategic Gatherings
    Keep workforce in the loop
    Engage for feedback and insights
  9. Newsletters from CEO

COMPACTS (Chapter Twelve)

A. Purpose: create an explicit written commitment for you and your partners
B. Considerations
  1. Explicit and enduring
  2. Not a contract

PART THREE – SYSTEMS

LANGUAGE (Chapter Thirteen)

A. Purpose: create an encompassing language focused on superior quality and the quality journey, and underscoring the shared mission and values that drive you

B. Considerations
1. Make quality your centerpiece
2. Attend and participate in new employee orientations
3. Schedule rounds where people work
4. Write regular newsletter or column
5. Join team or class where others participate away from workplace
6. Attend patient and employee funerals and special events
7. Demonstrate personal passions about patient care and superior quality
8. Conduct regular language audits
9. Use help from communications consultant/coach

LEARNING (Chapter Fourteen)

A. Purpose: create a culture that embraces learning focused on finding, implementing, improving, and inventing superior care solutions

B. Considerations
1. Measure care and care processes
2. Identify best care wherever you can find it outside organization
3. Use evidence-based analysis to establish performance boundaries
4. Language to support learning
5. Rewards and incentives to support learning
6. Report backs
7. Collaborative learning plans
8. Develop and maintain quality management expertise of senior leadership team, leadership network, and board of directors
9. Continuing education of all physicians and workforce in quality management, vision, and values
10. Metrics

TRANSPARENCY (Chapter Fifteen)

A. Purpose: create a "no secrets" culture to support learning and improvement

B. Considerations
1. With Patients

The patient covenant and promise (Bill of Rights)
Performance: About care
About performance
About preventable errors
About metrics
2. With Workforce
Performance
Issues and Decisions
3. With the Public
Performance
Involvement with you (let them see you at work)
Candor

INNOVATION (Chapter Sixteen)

A. Purpose: ensure that the organization maintains its lead in delivering the best care possible to those it serves through continuous improvement and innovation
B. Considerations
1. General
In-house v. Outside driven
Guided v. Spontaneous
2. Guiding Principles
Protection
Accountability
Support
Outside Expertise
Language
3. Organization
Visibility
Leadership
Funding

INFORMATION (Chapter Seventeen)

A. Purpose: provide pipes, reservoirs to store and move information to help clinical decisions, analyze performance, and assess improvement opportunities
B. Need: an overarching framework to guide
C. Focus Areas
1. Patients
Access to their personal information
Access to advice
On-line messaging with providers
On-line communications from providers and system

2. Clinicians

    Access to information and data required to diagnose and treat

    Access to work and decisions of team, and to communicate within the team and across teams

    Patient registries

    On-line order entry

    Evidence-based decision-support

    Real-time communications links to clinicians, support staff, and patients

3. Support Personnel

    Access to orders and communications from providers

    Two-way communications with clinicians and other staff

    Patient scheduling and tracking

4. System (Performance)

    Volume and use

    Quality

    Safety

    Service

    Costs

5. Improvement and Learning

6. Revenues and Billing

7. Regulatory and Legal compliance

D. Basic Rules

1. Keep it simple as possible

2. Fix processes first

3. Find solutions that fit your needs

4. Choose what you understand

5. Off-the-shelf where possible

6. Flexible and adaptable over time

7. Minimal customization

8. Carefully planned and adequately funded rollout

9. Budget for maintenance and upgrades

E. Oversight (The Steering Committee and CIO)

1. Oversee design and implementation

2. Generate Policy

3. Screen and recommend specific IT solutions

4. Review and approve customization request

5. Ensure data consistency and compatibility

6. Oversee analytic ("data mining") capabilities

PRODS (Chapter Eighteen)

A. Purpose: provoke organization to do what may be difficult, weaken resistance to change, and forestall returning to the past

B. Types
    1. Institutes
        Report to CEO
        Separately funded
        No operating responsibilities
        Credible leadership
        Independent board reporting to parent board
        Located in physician organization if clinical
        Outside funding to supplement
    2. Outside Consultants
        Finite engagements
        Strategy and issues vs. Ongoing operational responsibilities
        Senior and credible
        Contract and pay for value
        Adequate time to learn and grow
        Possible use to deliver bad news
        Connected with CEO throughout
    3. Other Outside Experts
        To review specific areas
        Recognized experts
        Visiting Committees
        Paid
        Permanent vs. Ad hoc
    4. Inside Experts
        Beware operating on the cheap
        Beware job expansions beyond bandwidth

ACCOUNTABILITY AND COMPENSATION (Chapter Nineteen)

  A. Purpose: reinforce values and strategies, and help attract and retain high quality professionals, managers, leaders, and support personnel
  B. Principles
    1. Design to meet your needs
    2. Change carefully and infrequently
    3. Emphasize and reward group and team performance
    4. Reinforce mission, values, and operating principles
    5. Provide significant feedback and coaching
    6. Value-based accountabilities instead of management by objectives
  C. Compensation Program
    1. Scope
        Salary
        "At Risk" compensation based on performance
        Benefits

   2. Structure

      Few pay bands with separation based on performance
        within bands

      Thirty to fifty organization comparator group to establish
        structure and maintain year-on-year stability

      Three to five organizations for qualitative comparisons

   3. Management

      Under CEO control

   4. Incentives

      Emphasize team, group, and department performance

      Allow each cluster to divide rewards among members
        consistent with principles you establish

      Establish reserve pool for special efforts and results

      Cash v. Non-Cash-Longevity v. Performance

      Should reward loyalty and perseverance

      Separate longevity and performance-related recognition

      Profit Sharing: graduated rewards capped at top and bottom

      Quality Gate: to establish all-or-nothing access to profit
        sharing or performance rewards

D. Traps

   1. The exception

   2. Money the only answer

   3. Slippery slope of "fixing" individual hiring and retention issues

OPERATING DISCIPLINE (Chapter Twenty)

A. Purpose: integrate your leadership, your partners, and your
   systems into a coherent engine of change

B. Characteristics

   1. Robust enough for the challenge

   2. Proven

   3. Reinforces mission and values

   4. Teachable and reproducible

   5. Analytical and data-driven

   6. Complements patient stories and expectations

   7. Focuses on day-to-day work of delivering care

   8. One not many

   9. Ubiquitous use

APPENDIX B:
CONTACTS

The following individuals gave generously of their time and insights:

Donald M. Berwick, MD: Founder, Institute for Healthcare Improvement, Cambridge, MA

Maureen A. Bisognano: President and CEO, Institute for Healthcare Improvement, Cambridge, MA

Richard M.J. Bohmer, MD: Professor, Management Practices, Harvard Business School, Harvard University, Cambridge, MA

Diane Cecchettini, RN: President and CEO, MultiCare Health System, Tacoma, WA

Alan Channing: President and CEO, Sinai Health System, Chicago, IL

Molly J. Coye, MD: Chief Innovation Officer, UCLA Health, Los Angeles, CA

James A. Diegel: President and CEO, St. Charles Health System, Bend, OR

Michael J. Dowling: President and CEO, North Shore-LIJ Health System, Manhasset, NY

Susan Edgman-Levitan, PA: Executive Director, John D. Stoeckle Center for Primary Care Innovation, Massachusetts General Hospital, Boston, MA

David T. Feinberg, MD: Assoc. Vice Chancellor, President, & CEO, UCLA Health, Los Angeles, CA

Teri G. Fontenot: President and CEO, Woman's Hospital, Baton Rouge, LA

Patricia A. Gabow, MD: Chief Executive Officer, Denver Health, Denver, CO

Dean Gruner, MD: President & CEO, ThedaCare, Appleton, WI

John Horty: Chairman, Horty, Springer, & Mattern, PC, Pittsburgh, PA

Brent C. James, MD: Chief Quality Officer & Executive Director, Institute for Health Care Delivery Research, Intermountain Healthcare, Salt Lake City, UT

Maulik S. Joshi, DrPH: President, Health Research & Educational Trust, Chicago, IL

Gary S. Kaplan, MD: Chairman & CEO, Virginia Mason Health System, Seattle, WA

Arnold Milstein, MD: Director, Stanford Clinical Excellence Research Center, Palo Alto, CA

Ian Morrison, PhD: Healthcare Futurist, Palo Alto, CA

Philip A. Newbold: Chief Executive Officer, Beacon Health System, South Bend, IN

John O'Brien: Former President & CEO, UMass Memorial Health Care, Worcester, MA

Paul H. O'Neill: Former Secretary of the US Treasury and Former CEO Alcoa Aluminum, Pittsburgh, PA

Marc E. Owen (and team): President, McKesson Specialty Health, San Francisco, CA

Ronald A. Paulus, MD: President & CEO, Mission Health, Asheville, NC

Judy Rich (and team): President & CEO, TMC HealthCare, Tucson, AZ

Sara J. Singer: Associate Professor of Health Care Management and Policy, School of Public Health, Harvard University, Cambridge, MA

Mark D. Smith, MD: President & CEO, California HealthCare Foundation, Oakland, CA

Glenn D. Steele, Jr., MD: President & CEO, Geisinger Health System, Danville, PA

Ross E. Stromberg: Director, PricewaterhouseCoopers, Healdsburg, CA

John Toussaint, MD. Chief Executive Officer, ThedaCare Center for Healthcare Value, Appleton, WI

Richard J. Umbdenstock: President & CEO, American Hospital Association, Washington, DC

A. Eugene Washington, MD: Vice Chancellor, UCLA Health Sciences, Los Angeles, CA

Stephen A. Williams: Chief Executive Officer, Norton Healthcare, Louisville, KY

Nicholas Wolter, MD: Chief Executive Officer, Billings Clinic, Billings, MT

Bibliography

Altman, Stuart and David Shactman. *Power, Politics, and Universal Health Care*. Amherst, NY: Prometheus Books, 2011

Anderson, Avis H. *A&P: The Story of the Great Atlantic and Pacific Tea Company*. Mount Pleasant, SC: Arcadia Publishing, 2002

Barken, Frederick M., MD. *Out of Practice: Fighting for Primary Care Medicine in America*. Ithaca, NY: Cornell University Press, 2011

Barnes, Julian. *The Sense of an Ending*. New York: Alfred A. Knopf, 2011

Berwick, Donald M. *Escape Fire: Designs for the Future of Health Care*. San Francisco: Jossey-Bass, 2007

Bisognano, Maureen, and Charles Kenney. *Pursuing the Triple Aim: Seven Innovators Show the Way to Better Care, Better Health, and Lower Costs*. San Francisco: Jossey-Bass, 2012

Bloche, M. Gregg, MD. *The Hippocratic Myth: Why Doctors are Under Pressure to Ration Care, Practice Politics, and Compromise Their Promise to Heal*. New York: Palgrave Macmillan, 2011

Bohmer, Richard, M. J. *Designing Care: Aligning the Nature and Management of Health Care*. Cambridge: Harvard Business Review Press, 2009

Burns, Lawton Robert, ed. *The Business of Healthcare Innovation, Second Edition*. Cambridge: Cambridge University Press, 2012

Calico, Forrest, with Joyce Sweeney Martin. *Out of the Blue: How Open Doors and Unexpected Paths Set the Course of My Life* (Bloomington, IN: CrossBooks, 2012)

Carroll, Paul B. and Chunka Mui. *Billion Dollar Lessons: What You Can Learn from the Most Inexcusable Business Failures of the Last 25 Years*. New York: Penguin, 2008

Charan, Ram. *Boards That Deliver: Advancing Corporate Governance from Compliance to Competitive Advantage*. San Francisco: Jossey-Bass, 2007

Christensen, Clayton M., Jerome H. Grossman, MD, and Jason Hwang, MD. *The Innovator's Prescription: A Disruptive Solution for Health Care*. New York: McGraw-Hill, 2008

Cosgrove, Delos M., Michael Fisher, Patricia Gabow, Gary Gottlieb, George C. Halvorson, Brent C. James, Gary S. Kaplan, Jonathan B. Perlin, Robert Petzel, Glenn D. Steel, and John S. Toussaint. "Ten Strategies to Lower Costs, Improve Quality, and Engage Patients: The View from Leading Health System CEOs" *Health Affairs* 32, no. 2 (2013):321-327

Crosson, Francis J., and Laura A. Tollen. *Partners in Health: How Physicians and Hospitals Can Be Accountable Together*. San Francisco: Jossey-Bass, 2010

Drucker, Peter F. *Managing the Nonprofit Organization: Principles and Practices*. New York: HarperBusiness, 1990, reprinted 2006

De Pree, Max. *Leadership Jazz - Revised Edition: The Essential Elements of a Great Leader*. New York: Crown Business/Random House, reprint 2008

Duhigg, Charles. *The Power of Habit: Why We Do What We Do in Life and Business*. New York: Random House, 2012

Enthoven, Alain C., and Laura A Tollen, eds. *Toward a 21st Century Health System: The Contributions and Promise of Prepaid Group Practice*. San Francisco: Jossey-Bass, 2004

Enzmann, Dieter F. *Surviving in Health Care*. St. Louis: Mosby, 1997

Fogg, B.J., and Dean Eckles, eds. *Mobile Persuasion: 20 Perspectives on the Future of Behavior Change*. Stanford: Stanford Captology Media, 2007

Frisina, Michael E. *Influential Leadership: Change Your Behavior, Change Your Organization, Change Health Care*. Chicago: AHA Press, 2011

Gardner, Karen, ed. *Better CEO-Board Relations: Practical Advice for a Successful Partnership*. Chicago: AHA Press, 2007

Gardner, Karen, ed. *The Excellent Board II: New, Practical Solutions for Health Care Trustees and CEOs*. Chicago: AHA Press, 2008

Gawande, Atul. *Better: A Surgeon's Notes on Performance*. New York: Metropolitan Books, 2007

Gawande, Atul. "Cowboys and Pit Crews." *The New Yorker* May 21, 2011, http://www.newyorker.com/online/blogs/newsdesk/2011/05/atul-gawa-nde-harvard-medical-school-commencement-address.html

Geyman, John. *Breaking Point: How the Primary Care Crisis Endangers the Lives of Americans*. Friday Harbor, WA: Copernicus Healthcare, 2011

Goodwin, Doris Kearns. *Team of Rivals: The Political Genius of Abraham Lincoln*. New York: Simon & Schuster, 2006

Groopman, Jerome, MD. *How Doctors Think*. Boston-New York: Houghton Mifflin Harcourt, 2008

Halvorson, George C. *Health Care Reform Now! A Prescription for Change*. San Francisco: Jossey-Bass, 2007

Halvorson, George C. *Health Care Will Not Reform Itself: A User's Guide to Refocusing and Reforming American Health Care*. Boca Raton: Productivity Press/CRC Press, 2009

Halvorson, George C. *KP Inside: 101 Letters to the People of Kaiser Permanente*. CreateSpace Independent Publishing Platform, 2012

Ham, Chris, Judith Smith, and Elizabeth Eastmure. *Commissioning integrated care in a liberated NHS: Research Summary*. London: Nuffield Trust, 2011

Hammes, Bernard J., PhD, ed. *Having Your Own Say: Getting the Right Care When it Matters Most*. Washington, DC: CHT Press, 2012

Holsinger, James W., ed. *Contemporary Public Health: Principles, Practice, and Policy*. Lexington: The University Press of Kentucky, 2012

Iansiti, Marco, and Roy Levien. *The Keystone Advantage: What the New Dynamics of Business Ecosystems Mean for Strategy, Innovation, and Sustainability*. Cambridge: Harvard Business Review Press, 2004

Institute of Medicine. "A CEO Checklist for High-Value Health Care," discussion paper authored by Delos M. Cosgrove, Michael Fisher, Patricia Gabow, Gary Gottlieb, George C. Halvorson, Brent C. James, Gary S. Kaplan, Jonathan B. Perlin, Robert Petzel, Glenn D. Steel, and John S. Toussaint. Washington, DC: IOM Roundtable on Value & Science-Driven Health Care, 2012

Institute of Medicine. "Crossing the Quality Chasm: A New Health System for the 21st Century," A Report from the Committee on the Quality of Health Care in America, Washington, DC: National Academy Press, 2001

Institute of Medicine. *Informing the Future, Sixth Edition*. Washington, DC: 2011

Institute of Medicine. *To Err is Human: Building a Safer Health System*, edited by Linda T. Kohn, Janet M. Corrigan, and Molla S. Donaldson. Washington, DC: National Academies Press, 2000

Johnson, Steven. *Where Good Ideas Come From: The Natural History of Innovation*. New York: Riverhead Trade, 2010, reprint 2011

Joshi, Maulik S., and Bernard J. Horak. *Healthcare Transformation: A Guide for the Hospital Board Member*. Boca Raton: Productivity Press/ CRC Press, 2009

Kahneman, Daniel. *Thinking, Fast and Slow*. New York: Farrar, Straus and Giroux, 2011

Kenagy, John. *Designed to Adapt: Leading Healthcare in Challenging Times*. Bozeman, MT: Second River Healthcare, 2009

Kenney, Charles. *The Best Practice: How the New Quality Movement is Transforming Medicine*. New York: PublicAffairs, 2008

Kenney, Charles. *Transforming Health Care: Virginia Mason Medical Center's Pursuit of the Perfect Patient Experience*. Boca Raton: CRC Press, 2010

Kochan, Thomas A., Adrienne E. Eaton, Robert B. McKersie, and Paul S. Adler. *Healing Together: The Labor-Management Partnership at Kaiser Permanente*. Ithaca and London: ILR Press, 2009

James, Brent C., and Lucy A Savitz. "How Intermountain trimmed health care costs through robust quality improvement effort." *Health Affairs* 30 no. 6, 2011:1185-91

Kotkin, Joel. The Next Hundred Million: America in 2050. New York: Penguin Press, 2010

Kotter, John P. A Sense of Urgency. Boston: Harvard Business Press, 2008

Kotter, John P., and Dan S. Cohen. *The Heart of Change: Real-Life Stories of How People Change Their Organizations*. Boston: Harvard Business Review Press, 2012

Kotter, John P. *Leading Change*. Boston: Harvard Business Review Press, 1996, new preface 2012

Kumar, Sanjaya, MD, and David B. Nash, MD. *Demand Better! Revive Our Broken Healthcare System*. Bozeman, MT: Second River Healthcare, 2010

Lauer, Charles. *Decency*. Bozeman, MT: Second River Healthcare, 2005

Lawrence, David. *From Chaos to Care: The Promise of Team-Based Medicine*. Cambridge: Perseus Publishing/De Capo Press, 2002

Lawrence, David. "My Mother and the Medical Ad-Hoc-Racy." *Health Affairs* 22 no. 3, 2003:238-242

Lee, Fred. *If Disney Ran Your Hospital: 9 1/2 Things You Would Do Differently*. Bozeman, MT: Second River Healthcare, 2004

Leebov, Wendy. *Wendy Leebov's Essentials for Great Patient Experiences: No-Nonsense Solutions with Gratifying Results*. Chicago: Health Forum/ AHA Press, 2008

Lerner, Josh. *Boulevard of Broken Dreams: Why Public Efforts to Boost Entrepreneurship and Venture Capital Have Failed – and What to Do About It*. Princeton: Princeton University Press, 2009

Levey, Gerald S., MD. *Never Be Afraid to Do the Right Thing*. (Bozeman, MT: Second River Healthcare, 2011

Loch, Christoph H., Stephen Chick, and Arnd Huchzermeier. *Management Quality and Competitiveness: Lessons from the Industrial Excellence Award*. Berlin: Springer, 2008

Ludmerer, Kenneth M. *Time to Heal: American Medical Education from the Turn of the Century to the Era of Managed Care*. Oxford: Oxford University Press USA, 1999, reprint 2005

Marmor, Theodore R., Richard Freeman, and Kieke G. H. Okma, eds. *Comparative Studies and the Politics of Modern Medical Care*. New Haven: Yale University Press, 2009

Marmot, Michael. *The Status Syndrome: How Social Standing Affects Our Health and Longevity*. New York: Holt Paperbacks, 2005

Michelli, Joseph A. *Prescription for Excellence: Leadership Lessons for Creating a World-Class Customer Experience from UCLA Health System*. New York: McGraw-Hill; Bozeman, MT: Second River Healthcare, 2011

Millard, Candace. *The River of Doubt: Theodore Roosevelt's Darkest Journey*. New York: Broadway Books, 2006

Morrison, Ian. *Leading Change in Health Care: Building a Viable System for Today and Tomorrow*. Chicago: Health Forum/AHA Press, 2011

Mullan, Fitzhugh, Ellen Ficklen, and Kyna Rubin. *Narrative Matters: The Power of the Personal Essay in Health Policy*. Baltimore: The Johns Hopkins University Press, 2006

Mulley, Albert G., Chris Trimble, and Glyn Elwyn. *Patients' Preferences Matter: Stop the Silent Misdiagnosis*. London: The Kings Fund, 2012

Nance, John J., and Kathleen M. Bartholomew. *Charting the Course: Launching Patient-Centric Healthcare.* Bozeman, MT: Second River Healthcare, 2012

Nance, John J. *Why Hospitals Should Fly: The Ultimate Flight Plan to Patient Safety and Quality Care.* Bozeman, MT: Second River Healthcare, 2008

National Academy of Engineering and Institute of Medicine. *Building a Better Delivery System: A New Engineering/Health Care Partnership.* Edited by Proctor P. Reid, W. Dale Compton, Jerome H. Grossman, and Gary Fanjiang. Washington, DC: The National Academies Press, 2005

Newbold, Philip A., and Diane Serbin Stover. *Wake Up and Smell the Innovation! Stirring Up a Return on Imagination.* Chicago: Networlding Publishing, 2011

Nolte, Ellen, and Martin McKee. *Caring for People with Chronic Conditions: A Health System Perspective.* Berkshire, England: Open University Press, 2008

Pink, Daniel H. *Drive: The Surprising Truth about What Motivates Us.* New York: Riverhead Books, 2009

Pointer, Dennis D. *Navigating the Boardroom: 40 Maxims, Things You Must Know and Do to Be a Great Director.* Bozeman, MT: Second River Healthcare, 2008

Porter, Roy. *The Greatest Benefit to Mankind: A Medical History of Humanity.* New York: W. W. Norton & Company, 1999

Prybil, Lawrence, Samuel Levey, Rex Killian, David Fardo, Richard Chait, David Bardach, and William Roach. "Governance in Large Nonprofit Health Systems: Current Profile and Emerging Patterns." Lexington, KY; Commonwealth Center for Governance Studies, Inc, 2012, http://www.mc.uky.edu/publichealth/documents/Governance_booklet_FINAL.pdf

Reid, T. R. *The Healing of America: A Global Quest for Better, Cheaper, and Fairer Health Care.* New York: Penguin, 2010

Rockefeller Foundation, The. "Pocantico II: The Global Challenge of Health Systems." New York, The Rockefeller Foundation, 2007

Rose, Geoffrey, with comments by Michael Marmot and Kay-Tee Khaw. *Rose's Strategy of Preventive Medicine.* Oxford: Oxford University Press USA, updated 2008

Scott, Mark, and Leland Kaiser, with Richard Baltus. *Courage to Be First: Becoming the First Planetree Hospital in America.* Bozeman, MT: Second River Healthcare, 2009

Scutchfield, F. Douglas, and C. William Keck. *Principles of Public Health Practice, Third Edition.* Stamford, CT: Cengage Learning, 2009

Senor, Dan, and Saul Singer. *Start-Up Nation: The Story of Israel's Economic Miracle.* New York and Boston: Twelve, 2009

Shortell, Stephen M., Robin R. Gillies, David A. Anderson, Karen Morgan Erickson, and John B. Mitchell. *Remaking Health Care in America: The Evolution of Organized Delivery Systems.* San Francisco: Jossey-Bass, 2000

Smith, Judith, and Jennifer Dixon. "Can NHS Hospitals Do More With Less?" London: Nuffield Trust, 2012

Spath, Patrice L., ed. *Engaging Patients as Safety Partners: A Guide for Reducing Errors and Improving Satisfaction.* Chicago: Health Forum/ AHA Press, 2008

Starr, Paul. *The Social Transformation of American Medicine: The Rise of a Sovereign Profession and the Making of a Vast Industry.* New York: Basic Books, 1982

Thorndike, William N. *The Outsiders: Eight Unconventional CEOs and Their Radically Rational Blueprint for Success.* Boston: Harvard Business Review Press, 2012

Toussaint, John, and Roger Gerard. *On the Mend: Revolutionizing Healthcare to Save Lives and Transform the Industry.* Cambridge: Lean Enterprise Institute, 2010

Toussaint, John, with Emily Adams. *Potent Medicine: The Collaborative Cure for Healthcare.* Appleton, WI: ThedaCare Center for Healthcare Value, 2012

Vogel, Ezra F. *Deng Xiaoping and the Transformation of China.* Cambridge, MA: The Belknap Press of Harvard University Press, 2011

Walsh, Diana. (President Emerita) "Educating Our Smartest Kids to Tackle the Big Problems in Healthcare" Wellesley College, May 18, 2013

Whitman, Steven, Ami M. Shah, and Maureen R. Benjamins, eds. *Urban Health: Combating Disparities with Local Data.* Oxford: Oxford University Press, 2011

Yih, Yuehwern, ed. *Handbook of Healthcare Delivery Systems.* Boca Raton: CRC Press, 2011

About the Author

Dr. Lawrence served as CEO and chairman of Kaiser Foundation Health Plan and Hospitals until his retirement in 2002. He was appointed CEO in 1991 and chairman the next year. He currently pursues interests in new business development, teaching, public policy, and writing. He is a member of the boards of Agilent Technologies, McKesson Corporation, Proteus Digital Health, Aditazz, and Cellworks. He is a member of the Health Advisory Boards of the RAND Corporation; an advisor to the CEOs of SomaLogic, Inc., MedExpert, Inc., and TangramCare; associated with Artiman Ventures, and teaches with the Estes Park Institute. He consults with selected healthcare systems that pursue advanced integration strategies.

Prior to joining Kaiser Permanente in 1981, Dr. Lawrence worked in Public Health and Human Services in Multnomah County, OR; on the faculty of the University of Washington School of Public Health and Community Medicine and the School of Medicine; as an advisor to the Ministry of Health of Chile; and as a Peace Corps Physician.

Dr. Lawrence is a founding board member of the Lucian Leape Institute of the National Patient Safety Foundation and a Distinguished Advisor to the NPSF. He is a member of the Institute of Medicine and the AOA physician honor society. He is the author of *From Chaos to Care: The Promise of Team-Based Medicine* (Perseus, 2002).

Dr. Lawrence received his bachelor's degree from Amherst College (1962), his MD from the University of Kentucky (1966), his Masters of Public Health from the University of Washington (1973). He completed his Residency in General Preventive Medicine at Johns Hopkins University and the University of Washington, and is Board Certified in

General Preventive Medicine (1974). He has received honorary degrees from Amherst College, University of Kentucky, and Cornell University, and is a member of the University of Kentucky Alumni Hall of Fame and the University of Kentucky College of Public Health Hall of Fame.

He is married to the former Stephanie Ann Poche. They have four children and seven grandchildren, and divide their time between Geyserville, CA, and Black Butte Ranch, OR.